MW01493267

RICHARD H. RAHE, M.D.

PATHS TO HEALTH AND RESILIENCE

Copyright © 2009 Richard H. Rahe, M.D.
All rights reserved.

ISBN: 1-4392-4905-9
ISBN-13: 9781439249055

Visit www.booksurge.com to order additional copies.

Paths to Health and Resilience

Manage Stress and Build Coping

Richard H. Rahe, M.D.

Health Assessment Programs, Inc.

Table of Contents

Table of Contents   page v

List of Illustrations   page vi

List of Tables   page vii

Introduction   page ix

Who You Are: First Stress Indicator   page 1

Recent Life Changes: Second Stress Indicator   page 9

Physical Symptoms: Third Stress Indicator   page 17

Psychological Symptoms: Fourth Stress Indicator   page 25

Behaviors and Emotions: Fifth Stress Indicator   page 31

Your Total Stress Score   page 39

Health Habits: First Coping Indicator   page 41

Social Support: Second Coping Indicator   page 47

Responses to Stress: Third Coping Indicator   page 53

Life Satisfactions: Fourth Coping Indicator   page 65

Purpose and Connections: Fifth Coping Indicator   page 73

Your Total Coping Score   page 81

Balance between Stress and Coping   page 83

Stress and Coping Relationship Graph   page 85

Summary and Permissions   page 87

Group Instructions   page 93

List of Illustrations

Figure 1.   **Your Strengths of Character**   page   3

Figure 2.   **Social Support Exercise**   page 50

Figure 3.   **Bound and Painfully Stretched**   page 56

Figure 4.   **Writing Notes to Later Hide**   page 57

Figure 5.   **The Tap Code**   page 58

Figure 6.   **Tapping and Receiving Code**   page 59

Figure 7.   **Stress and Coping Relationship**   page 85

List of Tables

Table 1.   **Who You Are Questions**   page 6

Table 2.   **Stress Totals for Who You Are**   page 7

Table 3.   **Life Changes Units I**   page 10

Table 4.   **Life Changes Units II**   page 11

Table 5.   **Life Changes Units III**   page 12

Table 6.   **Recent Life Changes Questions**   page 15

Table 7.   **Stress Totals for Recent Life Changes**   page 16

Table 8.   **Physical Symptoms Questions**   page 22

Table 9.   **Stress Totals for Physical Symptoms**   page 23

Table 10.   **Psychological Symptoms Questions**   page 28

Table 11.   **Stress Totals for Psychological Symptoms** page 29

Table 12.   **Behaviors and Emotions Questions**   page 37

Table 13.   **Stress Totals for Behaviors and Emotions** page 38

Table 14.   **Your Total Stress Score**   page 39

Table 15.   **Health Habits Questions**   page 42

Table 16.   **Coping Totals for Health Habits**   page 42

Table 17.   **Social Support Questions**   page 47

Table 18.   **Coping Totals for Social Supports**   page 47

Table 19.   **Responses to Stress Questions**   page 62

Table 20.   **Coping Totals for Responses to Stress**   page 62

Table 21.   **Life Satisfactions Questions**   page 66

Table 22.   **Coping Totals for Life Satisfactions**   page 66

Table 23. **Purpose and Connection Questions**   page 74

Table 24. **Coping Totals for Purpose and Connection** page 74

Table 25. **Your Total Coping Score**   page 81

Introduction

Persons using the words "stress," "coping," and "resilience," usually don't explain what they mean. The word stress, for example, is often used for life challenges ranging from a minor annoyance to a major catastrophe. Coping is often used to describe someone "holding up" under stress. How such coping is accomplished is rarely specified. Resilience is a word frequently used to describe persons "bouncing back" from stress. In modern medicine, these words are far more specific. The term stress generally refers to very significant life difficulties and challenges. Coping most often describes various physical and psychological strategies that can help a person to reduce stress. Resilience is most often used to indicate a person's physical and psychological resources that help him or her deal with stress.

Stress, coping, and resilience are relatively new words in the field of medicine, but earlier concepts go back several hundreds of years. Paul Rosch, M.D., President of the American Institute of Stress, has noted that Galen and Aesculapius, both early Greek physicians, discovered that demanding life events aroused "passions and perturbations of the soul." Rosch further noted that Moses Maimonides, the famous physician to the Sultan of Egypt, wrote, "[P]assions of the psyche produce changes in the body that are great...evident and manifest to all." Centuries later, Shakespeare, in his famous plays, frequently portrayed challenging life situations in the lives of his characters that brought forth serious mental and physical disorders.

In the nineteenth century, the field of medicine developed a strong biological emphasis when bacteria were discovered to cause some illnesses. Microscopes shifted the focus away from stress and onto observations made in the laboratory. Sigmund Freud and his followers, however, continued to emphasize the role of traumatic life events in persons' lives that could lead to major illnesses. British and American doctors engaged in the two World Wars of the twentieth century published observations on soldiers experiencing combat stresses with subsequent deleterious effects on their physical and mental health. Studies of life stress and illness over the most recent fifty years have established that stress is often an important contributing cause for a wide variety of illnesses, including coronary heart disease, cancer, arthritis, diabetes, and AIDS.

Measures of Stress and Coping

My first studies of stress and illness began when I was a medical student working with Professor Thomas H. Holmes, M.D., who was a specialist in internal medicine. During my postgraduate training in both psychiatry and internal medicine, I worked with Dr. Holmes to develop a scale that measured varying intensities of forty-three life stress events representative of common demands in a person's work, home and family, social and community relationships, and finances. From these early studies, and through further investigations I carried out in the U.S. Navy, it became evident that the higher the number and severities of one's recent life stresses over the previous year the more likely it was that they would experience an illness during the following year. Persons with extremely high recent life stress intensities tended to develop the most severe illnesses and/or injuries.

As my research career progressed, I found stress indicators other than recent life changes were also valuable explanations of a person's vulnerabilities to illness. These stress indicators included difficult early childhood experiences, current physical and psychological illnesses, and selected behaviors and emotions leading to anger, aggression, self-sacrifice, and despair. I therefore created an inventory that measured four stress indicators along with four measures of coping. My coping indicators were: diet and exercise; social support; helpful responses to stress; and life satisfactions. I called this instrument the Stress and Coping Inventory, or SCI.

The SCI proved to be very successful, especially in a large-scale study that I conducted in San Jose, California, in the 1990s. This study was designed to see if improvement in workers' health could be achieved through an educational program based on the SCI. Over five hundred employees were randomly divided into three groups. The first group, given the label "full intervention," was provided six, ninety-minute, biweekly group educational sessions. During these sessions, subjects utilized feedback from their initial SCI, as well as additional information from me and my co-therapist. Educational sessions for the full intervention group closely resemble what I present in this book.

The second group, given the label "partial intervention," received no group educational sessions but did receive feedback from their initial SCI results by mail. The third group, assigned as "control subjects," received no educational sessions and no SCI feedback information until the end of the study where they were received SCI feedback from their initial, mid-year, and year-end testing by mail and were offered a single educational session. At the end of the year-long study, subjects' medical records were reviewed for all doctor visits over the study year. The full intervention group showed **34% fewer doctor visits** than did subjects assigned the other two groups.

As helpful as the SCI proved to be in this study, it took thirty to forty-five minutes for persons to complete it. Therefore, I shortened and revised the SCI, added one additional stress indicator (looking at feelings of helplessness and hopelessness) and one more coping measure (purpose and meaning in life) and named it the Brief

Stress and Coping Inventory, or BSCI. The BSCI takes only ten to fifteen minutes to complete and is the basis of this book. A separate chapter is written for each of the five stress indicators and for each of the five coping modalities of the BSCI. A final chapter examines the reader's current balance between stress and coping in their lives, and provides them with measures of their near-future illness risk versus their resilience against illness.

Instructions for Scoring the BSCI

As you read each chapter in this book, you will be asked to mark those questions that apply to you concerning your current stresses and coping skills. You are then instructed to go back and sum the numbers found next to each question that you marked. The sum of all these numbers in a chapter is called your *Chapter Total*.

For the five Stress Indicator chapters you should next find the table titled *Stress Totals.* This table presents four *Categories of Responses.* Your Chapter Total will fall into one of the four Categories of Responses. From your Category of Responses you will see the number of *Stress Points* that your Chapter Total is given. These points will range from 0 to 3. Last, write your number of Stress Points in the space indicated near the end of the chapter. If you don't want to mark your book, use a sheet of scratch paper to record your points as you progress through the book.

For the five Coping Indicator chapters you will find a table titled *Coping Totals* containing four *Categories of Responses.* From this table, you will find the number of *Coping Points* that your Chapter Total is given. Write your number of Coping Points in the space found near the end of the chapter, or on your sheet of scratch paper.

In the middle of the book, you will calculate your *Total Stress Score* by adding all of your Stress Points from the five stress indicator chapters. Near the end of the book, you will similarly calculate your *Total Coping Score* by adding all your Coping Points from the five coping chapters. You can then plot your balance between stress and coping by finding where these two total scores intersect on the *Stress and Coping Relationship* graph. From this graph, you will see whether or not you are at risk for near-future illness. If you are at risk, the amount of risk will also be made clear on the graph. If you are not at risk, you will be able to assess your amount of resilience against near-future illnesses.

Intended Audiences for this Book

This BSCI workbook was devised for adults, from teenage years to senior status, for them to discover their current levels of life stress and coping skills. By working on stress management suggestions and building their coping skills they can reduce their near-future illness risk and increase their resilience. The BSCI, by itself, is found on my website www.drrahe.com.

Over the last few years, I have worked in three Veteran Affairs (VA) clinics specializing in treatment of current and former service men and women with post-traumatic stress disorder, or PTSD. You will read more about PTSD in the chapter entitled "Stress and Psychological Symptoms." I have been frustrated by not having sufficient time to provide these patients with a fuller understanding of how they can move from memories of combat stress on to analyzing and pursing the challenges of recovery that they face now that they have returned home. These challenges include reuniting with family members and friends, finding work, cutting back on alcohol and tobacco use, becoming a parent again, obtaining further education, and improving their finances. Therefore, I find these veterans are another audience for this book.

Further Information

Rosch, P. *Health and Stress; The Newsletter of the American Institute of Stress*. August, 2007.

Dubos, R. *Mirage of Health*. Harper and Row, New York, 1959.

Holmes, T.H. and Rahe, R.H. The Social Readjustment Rating Scale. *Journal of Psychosomatic Research*, 11:213-218, 1967.

Rahe, R.H. Epidemiological studies of life changes and illness. *International Journal of Psychiatry in Medicine*, 6(1/2):133-146, 1975.

Rahe, R.H., Taylor, C.B., Tolles, R.T., Newhall, L.M., Veach, T.V., and Bryson, S. A novel stress and coping workplace program reduces illness and health care utilization. *Psychosomatic Medicine*, 64:278-286, 2002.

Chapter 1: Who You Are

First Stress Indicator

Your Biological and Biographic Assets and Liabilities

Try not to be put off by the above title, which contains terminology that may sound more like what a tax accountant would use rather than a stress doctor. As you read further, you will begin to see the medical significances of this phrase, which has to do with resistances and vulnerabilities to illness starting from your conception to your present age. Liabilities are risks for illness and assets are resistances to illness. A risk doesn't mean definite trouble. It means possible trouble if a psychological or physical weakness is not recognized early and then carefully managed.

Let's start with some examples. Biological assets include genes inherited from our parents leading to long life and promoting high intelligence. Biological liabilities include parental genes that promote severe illnesses along with childhood and adult exposures to environmental toxins. Biographical assets include growing up in a stable and supportive household, receiving a good education, and learning to get along well with others. Biographical liabilities are the opposite of these assets.

Plentiful biological and biographic assets are a tremendous buffer against the development of physical and psychological illnesses across a lifetime. High numbers of biological and biographic liabilities, however, put you at risk for several physical and psychological illnesses, and when recognized should be modified if possible. For example, if a parent or grandparent died at an early age from coronary heart disease, you can reduce your risk for this illness by maintaining a healthy diet; engaging in regular physical

1

exercise; taking any needed medications, such as those for high blood pressure; and learning how to manage your life stresses.

Another example of modification of biological and biographical liabilities is seen for individuals who overcome disadvantages early in life to become successful later through their tenacity and hard work! I call overcoming liabilities in this manner "success through stress toughening."

Complete Your "Strengths of Character" Chart

Often overlooked as source of biographical assets are "gifts" that we received from parents, relatives, friends, and teachers during our early years. To identify such gifts, and their sources, I included my "Strengths of Character Chart" in this chapter. This chart uses a medical diagram originally devised to look for an inheritance pattern of major illnesses across generations. I changed this diagram to help you to track your gifts rather than family illnesses. See Figure 1.

To complete the chart, begin by writing the first names of your grandparents, parents, important aunts and uncles, and brothers and sisters next to the circles and squares that you find on the chart. Circles are for women and squares are for men. Add additional circles and squares to place other influential persons on the chart. (I'll tell you about lines for you and your spouse(s), if you are/were married, and for any children, later.)

Below each circle (for women) and square (for men) where you've written a name, see if you can remember one or two gifts that helped to develop your strength of character. For example, a grandfather may have shown you that pride in work leads to great life satisfactions. An aunt may have pointed out how you could discover reasons for a problem rather than simply being upset. It's likely that other relatives, teachers, and friends also gave you gifts. Note these gifts down below their names.

Your Strengths of Character

Your Strengths of Character will always be there to help you to manage severe stresses in your life! In this exercise review the strengths that you inherited, and were taught, by your family members. Also consider what you learned from important teachers, other adults, and peers.

Write the names of your family members in the circles (women) and squares (men). Near these circles and squares list the strengths they passed on to you - such as "honesty," "hard work," "trust," "compassion," etc. Do the same for influential aunts, uncles, teachers and other influential persons. List their "gifts" to you that helped to build your character.

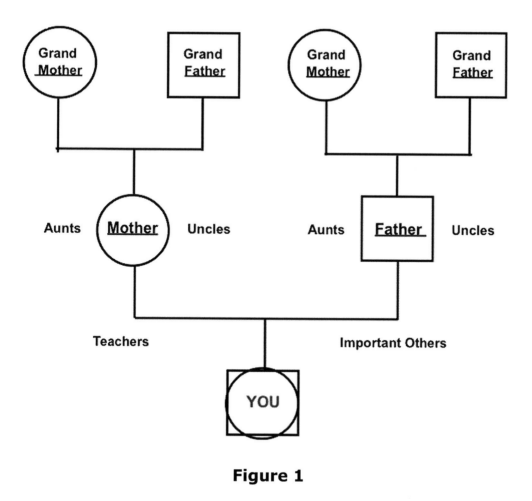

Figure 1

If married, fill in the name(s) of your spouse(es), and any children, by making new lines, circles, and squares on the chart. Children go below the line for you and your spouse(es). Some gifts skip generations. A child may think and behave more like one of your parents, or one of your grandparents, than you or your spouse. You may have been more influenced by a grandparent than a parent. A person outside your family, like a teacher or close friend, can often provide very important gifts to you as well. Be sure to put them in your chart.

What is the **best biographical asset** that you can have? I believe it is the experience of **successfully meeting and overcoming major life challenges.** Such success with challenges early in life very often promotes continuing successes throughout your later years. Review your completed chart and feel gratitude for your several gifts! We don't do this often enough! During major stressful situations, this is often a very helpful exercise.

When I was debriefing Americans held hostage in the American Embassy in Iran for sixteen months, many of them told me that they thought of their childhood years and it proved to be very helpful. The more they thought about this time in their lives, the more complete and vivid were their memories. Some mentioned that these recollections helped them learn how to be more patient, how to keep hope alive during severe stress, and encouraged them to help others in need.

One captive said that when he thought back over his early life, he first reflected on many negative situations that he had experienced with his father. Later, he began to see his father in a new light. He started to remember some positive things his father had done for him and the family, such as consistently providing money for food, clothing, and education. His father's punitive behaviors generally occurred after he had been drinking alcohol heavily. These negative experiences had previously clouded the positive aspects of his father. He said that he then began to forgive his father for his harsh punishments—essentially neutralizing this biographical liability.

Complete the BSCI "Who You Are" questions; find your Chapter Total and determine your Category of Responses

The BSCI "Who You Are" questions are listed in Table 1. As this is a stress indicator chapter your number and magnitude of selected biological and biographical liabilities are counted. Determine your Chapter Total for these questions, and then see where this total resides in the four Categories of Responses, shown in Table 2. From the Category where you find your Chapter Total, determine your "Who You Are" Stress Points (**Excellent** = 0 points; **Good** = 1 point; **Fair** = 2 points; **Worrisome** = 3 points) and write them in the space provided at the end of this chapter. If you don't want to mark your book, write them on a sheet of scratch paper.

Who You Are

				Male	Female
Asian	Hispanic Origin	White		Yes	No
Black	Native American	Other		Yes	No

Less than high school	High school graduate	Student	Retired
Some college/trade school	Associate degree	Semi-skilled	Skilled
College graduate	Graduate degree	Manager	Professional

Did you live with two parents (including stepparents)?	yes (0)	no (1)
Did your parents divorce or permanently separate?	yes (2)	no (0)
Did your mother die?	yes (2)	no (0)
Did your father die?	yes (2)	no (0)
Were you ever suspended from school?	yes (1)	no (0)
Were you ever arrested by the police?	yes (2)	no (0)
Did you have an alcohol and/or drug problem?	yes (3)	no (0)
Were you physically, sexually, and/or emotionally abused?	yes (3)	no (0)
		Total 1: _____

How often were your parents emotionally supportive?	Rarely (2)	Sometimes (1)	Often (0)
How often did your family (i.e. close relatives) get together?	Rarely (2)	Sometimes (1)	Often (0)
Did your family attend religious services?	Rarely (2)	Sometimes (1)	Often (0)
How often did your parents argue?	Rarely (0)	Sometimes (1)	Often (2)
Did you get good grades in school?	Rarely (2)	Sometimes (1)	Often (0)
Did you participate in school activities (including sports)?	Rarely (2)	Sometimes (1)	Often (0)
Did you date?	Rarely (2)	Sometimes (1)	Often (0)
Did you have a wide circle of friends?	Rarely (2)	Sometimes (1)	Often (0)
Did you have interesting hobbies (camping, crafts, music, collecting, etc.)?	Rarely (2)	Sometimes (1)	Often (0)
			Total 2: _____

Total 1 + Total 2: _____

Table 1

Stress Totals			
Chapter total:	**0 - 9**	**10 - 17**	**18 - 23**	**24 - 33**
Category:	**Excellent**	Good	Fair	**Worrisome**
Stress Points:	**Excellent 0,**	Good **1,**	Fair **2,**	**Worrisome 3**

Table 2

"Who You Are" Stress Points _____

Further Information

Waite, T. *Taken on Trust*. Harcourt Brace & Company, New York, 1993.

Tennant, C. Parental loss in childhood: Its effect in adult life. *Arch. Gen. Psychiatry*, 45:1045-1050, 1988.

Rahe, R.H., Karson, S., Howard, N.S., Rubin, R. T., and Poland, R.E. Psychological and physiological assessments on American hostages freed from captivity in Iran. *Psychosomatic Medicine*, 52:1-16, 1990.

Chapter 2: Recent Life Changes

Second Stress Indicator

Recent Life Changes

The development of the original Holmes and Rahe list of forty-three stressful life changes was mentioned in the previous chapter. In this chapter, the original list of life changes, along with their intensity ratings, will be compared with a duplicate list from a Miller and Rahe study carried out twenty-seven years later. Miller and Rahe discovered that average estimates for the intensities of these life changes had become significantly greater across the years. For example, a traffic ticket that was rated as 11 Life Change Units, or LCU, in 1967 was rated as 22 LCU in 1994.

Most of the lower rated LCU events in 1967 had more than doubled in intensity by the time of the second study. The higher rated LCU events in 1967 also increased in value by 20% to 30%. Averaging all LCU values from 1967 and comparing this average found in 1994, **life had become 44% more demanding** across these twenty-seven years. So if you have always thought that life is more difficult now than it was three decades ago, you are correct!

Below, Tables 3, 4, and 5 present the original list of forty-three life changes and their original LCU values, as well as the more recent LCU values for these life changes. You can see that every life change event increased in LCU value with the exception of marriage. The scaling method used required that one life change be arbitrarily assigned a LCU value thought to likely fall in the mid range of values. Marriage was the life change we selected and arbitrarily assigned it 50 LCU in both studies. Therefore, we have no idea as to LCU changes that may have occurred for marriage across these two studies.

Life Change Event	1967		1994	
	Rank	LCU	Rank	LCU
Death of Spouse	1	100	I	119
Divorce	2	73	2	98
Separation from Spouse	3	65	3	79
Jail Term	4	63	7	75
Death of Close Family Member	5	63	3	92
Major Personal Illness/Injury	6	53	6	77
Marriage	7	50	19	50
Fired from Work	8	47	5	79
Marital Reconciliation	9	45	13	57
Retirement	10	45	16	54
Major Illness in Family	11	44	14	56
Pregnancy	12	40	9	66
Sexual Difficulties	13	39	21	45
Gain New Family Member	14	39	12	57

Table 3

RECENT LIFE CHANGES: SECOND STRESS INDICATOR

Life Change Event	1967		1994	
	Rank	LCU	Rank	LCU
Major Business Adjustment	15	38	10	62
Major Financial Change	16	38	15	56
Death of Close Friend	17	37	8	70
Change Different Line of Work	18	36	17	51
Change in Spousal Arguments	19	35	18	51
Major Purchase	20	31	23	44
Financial Foreclosure	21	30	11	61
Change in Work Responsibility	22	29	24	43
Child Leaves Home	23	29	22	44
In-Law Troubles	24	29	28	38
High Personal Achievement	25	28	29	37
Spouse Begins or Stops Work	26	26	20	46
Begin or Cease Schooling	27	26	27	38
Change in Living Conditions	28	25	25	42

Table 4

Life Change Event	1967		1994	
	Rank	LCU	Rank	LCU
Change of Personal Habits	29	24	36	27
Troubles with Boss	30	23	33	29
Major Changes at Work	31	20	30	36
Change of Residence	32	20	26	41
Change to New School	33	20	31	35
Change in Recreation	34	19	34	29
Change in Church Activities	35	19	42	22
Change in Social Activities	36	18	38	27
Moderate Purchase	37	17	35	28
Change in Sleep Habits	38	16	40	26
Family Get-together Changes	39	15	39	26
Change in Eating Habits	40	15	37	27
Vacation	41	13	41	25
Christmas	42	12	32	30
Minor Violations of the Law	43	11	43	22
Average LCU values:		34	*and*	49

Table 5

Yearly LCU Totals Predict Illness Risk

In a large retrospective study I conducted before leaving my psychiatry residency, I discovered that persons reporting 0 to 100 LCU over the preceding year (in the mid 1960s) remained healthy over the following year. However, 30% of persons reporting 101 to 200 LCU the previous year reported a minor illness sometime during the next year. Fifty percent of individuals with life events totaling between 201 to 300 LCU over the prior year reported one or more minor illnesses, and occasionally a major illness, over the following year. Lastly, for persons reporting more than 300 LCU the previous year, 70% reported both minor and major illnesses across the next year. This study, along with later retrospective and prospective investigations that I carried out in the U.S. Navy, supported the observation that yearly LCU total values were predictive of risk for illness over the following year. The higher the initial LCU total, the greater the number of minor, severe, and even multiple illnesses that were reported across the next twelve months.

Complete the BSCI "Recent Life Changes" Questions

The number life changes that you will review in the BSCI questions that follow have increased to fifty-six. Over the years, I discovered that many life change events that were not chosen for the original study deserve to be included now. Newly added life changes include possible deaths of a child, parent, or sibling, as well as a close friend. These fifty-six life changes, and their most recently determined LCU values, are found in Table 6.

Circle, or make note of, the LCU number to the right of each life change that you experienced over the past year. The life change events are presented in two rows in the table due to the length of the list. Next, add all your circled LCU points (Total 1 plus Total 2) in Table 6. This is your Chapter Total LCU Score. In Table 7 find into which of the four Categories of Responses your Chapter Total is located. Once you have found the correct Category, you will see the number of Stress Points that apply. Write your Recent Life Changes Stress Points in the space provided near the end of this chapter, or make a note of these points on your scratch sheet.

RECENT LIFE CHANGES: SECOND STRESS INDICATOR

Recent Life Changes

Circle the number next to those events which happened to you <u>over the past year</u>.

Health

An illness or injury which was:

Very serious	74
Moderately severe	44
Less serious than above	20

Work

Change to a new type of work	51
Change in your work conditions	35
Change in work responsibilities	41
Taking courses to help you	18
Troubles at work	32
Major business readjustment	60
Loss of your job	74
Retirement	52

Home and Family

Change in residence	40
Major change in living conditions	42
Change in family get-togethers	25
Major change in health or behavior of a family member	55
Marriage	50
Pregnancy	67
Miscarriage or abortion	65
Birth (or adoption) of a child	66
Spouse begins or stops work	46
Change in arguments with spouse	50
Problems with relatives or in-laws	38
Parents dwivorce	59
Parent(s) remarry	50
Separation from spouse due to work or marital difficulties	79
Child leaves home	42

Home and Family, continued

Relative moves in with you	59
Divorce	96
Birth of grandchild	43
Death of spouse	119
Death of child	123
Death of parent or sibling	101

Personal and Social

Change in personal habits	26
Beginning or ending school	38
Change of school or college	35
Change in political beliefs	24
Change in religious beliefs	29
Change in social activities	27
Vacation	24
New, close, personal relationship	37
Engagement to marry	45
Personal relationship problems	39
Sexual difficulties	44
An accident	48
Minor violation of the law	20
Being held in jail	75
Major decision about your future	51
Major personal achievement	36
Death of a close friend	70

Financial

Major loss of income	60
Major increase in income	38
Loss of or damage to personal property	43
Major purchase	37
Minor purchase	20
Credit difficulties	56

Total of circled numbers 1: _____   Total of circled numbers 2: _____

Total 1 + Total 2:_____

Table 6

Stress Totals

Chapter Totals:	0 - 150	151 - 300	301 - 450	451+
Category:	Excellent	Good	Fair	Worrisome

As outlined above, place a **0, 1, 2,** or **3,** in the space next to **"Recent Life Changes" Stress Points** below, or on your scratch sheet.

Table 7

"Recent Life Changes" Stress Points _____

Further Information

Rahe, R.H. Life change measurement as a predictor of illness. *Proceedings of the Royal Society of Medicine*, 61:1124-1126, 1968.

Rahe, R.H. and Arthur, R.J. Life change patterns surrounding illness experience. *Journal of Psychosomatic Research*, 11:341-345, 1968.

Rahe, R.H., McKean, J.D., and Arthur, R.J. A longitudinal study of life change and illness patterns. *Journal of Psychosomatic Research*, 10:355-366, 1967.

Miller, M. and Rahe, R.H. Life changes scaling for the 1990s. *Journal of Psychosomatic Research*, 43:279-292, 1997.

Chapter 3: Physical Symptoms

Third Stress Indicator

One might initially believe that since recognition of life stress events, and their evaluations, take place in the brain, any resulting illnesses from stress would be "mental." Likewise, physical illnesses are generally thought to be the result of physical causes, such as inadequate diet, trauma, abnormal metabolism, and so forth. Such "physical causes" often explain illness vulnerability, but a person's perceptions and psychological reactions to life stress events help to explain the timing of onset and severity of physical illnesses.

Excellent examples of the effects of life stress in the timing of onset of coronary heart disease, the number one cause of death in the United States, were seen in a study I performed the late 1960s at the U.S. Naval Hospital In San Diego, California. I was a stress consultant to the Department of Medicine where I interviewed all men and women admitted to the hospital's Coronary Care Unit. Many of these patients were overweight, reported unhealthy diets, and didn't exercise regularly—so they showed illness vulnerability. When I inquired about possible recent life stresses, several patients became quite animated telling me about two or three such events. These patients were often convinced that these recent stresses were the immediate cause (timing of onset) of their heart attacks. Such stresses included significant problems at work, missing out on a promotion, marital and family issues, and financial setbacks.

These interviews influenced me to begin an early evening stress and coping program held at the Cardiology Clinic. Between six to eight patients comprised a group that met once a week over the first six weeks of their recovery. Each new group seemed to have the following three questions: "Why me?" (Why did I have a heart attack?); "Why now?" (Why did my heart attack occur at this time in my life?); and "What now?" (What can I do to recover and prevent another heart attack?).

Therefore, my initial group sessions dealt with the Why me and Why now questions. I began with discussions about vulnerability and the influences of genetics, gender, blood pressure, and diet. I moved on to topics of recent life stress. Typical life stresses included extensive overwork, impatience with delay, easily aroused anger and aggression, and rushing through life. Later sessions covered What now topics, including dietary changes, beginning consistent and moderate exercise, reducing overwork, controlling impatience, managing aggression, and finding solutions for many current life challenges.

The groups became very popular. To look for possible improved recovery resulting from these groups, I conducted a small study. Out of forty-four patients who were referred to my program, I randomly assigned half of them to my stress and coping groups and the other half to standard cardiac care. Medical reviews of the heart status for all patients could be obtained by review, once a year, of their military medical records. After four years of follow-up, patients receiving my educational sessions had developed significantly fewer new heart attacks, had experienced significantly fewer deaths from their disease, and had a significantly higher rate of return to work compared to those patients randomly assigned to standard coronary care.

Other researchers have later found similar benefits from group educational sessions for persons recovering from heart attacks. Even today, this approach remains valid. Unfortunately, managed care organizations do not pay medical practitioners to conduct such services. Only physicians and psychologists with research grants containing money for their salaries can continue this approach.

Following the publication of my stress and coping program for heart disease patients, I was awarded a National Institutes of Health Special Fellowship to leave active duty status with the

Navy for eighteen months and pursue further psychological studies of coronary heart disease patients at a hospital in Stockholm, Sweden that specialized in cardiology. With several Swedish co-investigators, I found once again that persons who had experienced a heart attack tended to recall a significant build-up of life stress events over the year or two preceding their attacks. Often, the year immediately prior to the attack was reported as the most stressful year of all. Recent studies by others have shown that if a patient recovering from a heart attack also suffers from psychological depression, his or her risk of developing another heart attack is further increased.

In another Swedish study, I examined the life stresses of patients who died suddenly from their coronary heart disease. Through interviews with the surviving spouses, I was able to learn the number and severity of life stresses the patients experienced over the two years leading up to their deaths. A second group of spouses whose husband or wife had survived a heart attack was used for comparison. Life stress events were found to be significantly higher in number, and higher in life change intensities, for sudden death victims than for the comparison group who survived their attacks. These results were later confirmed in much larger investigation carried out by researchers in Helsinki, Finland.

Precipitating versus Predisposing Stresses and Illness

Recent life stress events are considered to be *precipitating* factors of many illnesses. That is, the timing of a stressful event corresponds closely to the timing of the clinical onset of an illness. In contrast, long-term life stress influences on illness vulnerability are called *predisposing* factors. Do you remember the discussion from Chapter 1 about the lifelong effects of biographical liabilities (such as being a victim of abuse during childhood)? These can be predisposing factors for the onset of an illness.

Perhaps my most revealing study of the effects of predisposing factors on the development of coronary heart disease was also done while I was in Sweden. It was a study of the early life histories of sixty-four pairs of identical male twins, where one twin showed moderate to severe coronary heart disease while his twin brother was found to have little to no heart disease. These discordant twin pairs comprised only 15% of the entire twin sample under study. The other 85% of twin pairs proved to be nearly identical for their degrees of heart disease. Although the discordant twin pairs differed markedly in their degrees of heart disease, they had identical physical factors such as height, weight, blood chemistries, genetic markers, and so forth. After all, an identical twin pair is truly one person with two bodies. So my research question was: "Do these discordant twin pairs reveal important differences in predisposing life stresses?"

Swedish interviewers were kept unaware of the heart disease status of each twin they saw so not be biased by this knowledge as they recorded life history events. In reviewing these life histories for discordant twins, I knew which twin brother had the more severe heart disease and I found that the unhealthier twin brother was not as happy, and oftentimes depressed, compared to his healthier brother. Although physically inseparable, these twin pairs were not identical in how they had experienced and reacted to life challenges.

Here's an example pair of highly discordant twins. One twin brother was diagnosed as having experienced a previous heart attack and showed substantial current coronary heart disease while his twin brother had a perfectly normal cardiac exam. After reading my summaries of their early life histories below, can you tell which twin brother had the heart disease?

Twin #1 reported a happy childhood with many friends. He often invited friends to his home despite the fact that his grandfather was very senile and often roamed the house naked. Despite his behavior, Twin 1 liked his grandfather and his friends found the old man amusing. As the family was quite poor, his parents discouraged both children from attending university, despite the fact that both of them had done very well in their early schooling. Searching for jobs where a higher education was not a requirement, Twin #1 became a forest ranger. He reported that he thoroughly enjoyed his job, especially walking alone in the woods out in nature.

Twin #2 also reported that his family was quite poor, and because of that he was deprived of many things, including the chance to attend a university. He emphasized to the interviewer that he would have excelled at a university based on his prior performance in his early schooling. He avoided playing with other children and had few friends. He never invited anyone to his house as his grandfather was an embarrassment to him. He disliked his current job, believing it was beneath his skills and potential. He repeatedly blamed his lack of higher education as the main cause of his generally unsatisfactory life.

I'm sure you didn't need to guess. As environmental influences (home, parents, family, diet, and so forth) were essentially the same for these twin brothers, their differing life satisfactions were most likely due to differences in their perceptions and reactions to their life stresses starting in early childhood. The healthier brother met with poverty, his grandfather's senility, his lack of higher education, and a limited job choice with apparent acceptance and little regret. In contrast, his unhealthy brother appeared to never have made such adjustments to these life challenges and carried his reported early unhappiness throughout his adult life.

Complete the BSCI "Physical Symptoms" Questions

Answer the questions in Table 8 below. If you previously discovered that your recent life changes from the previous chapter were high, you may now find that your number of current physical symptoms of illnesses is also high. This would be another example of high life changes precipitating an elevation of physical symptoms of illness. In contrast, if you recorded very few recent life changes you may likely have marked very few physical illness symptoms.

Physical Symptoms

Indicate whether you have experienced any of the following conditions <u>over the past year</u>.

Respiratory			Musculoskeletal		
Have you suffered from a stuffy nose?	yes	no	Have your muscles been stiff or painful?	yes	no
Has your throat been sore or infected?	yes	no	Were you bothered by back pain?	yes	no
Did you have asthma or hay fever?	yes	no	Did you have tension headaches?	yes	no
Gastrointestinal			**Neurological**		
Was your stomach frequently upset?	yes	no	Did you suffer from migraine headaches?	yes	no
Was constipation or diarrhea a problem?	yes	no	Did you have numbness or tingling?	yes	no
Were hemorrhoids a problem?	yes	no	Have you had dizzy spells?	yes	no
Cardiovascular			**Genitourinary**		
Did you have high blood pressure?	yes	no	Were there kidney or bladder problems?	yes	no
Has your heartbeat been irregular?	yes	no	Women: menstrual difficulties?	yes	no
Have you had any heart pain?	yes	no	Men: prostate problems?	yes	no
General Health			**Dermatological**		
Were you under or overweight?	yes	no	Did your skin itch frequently?	yes	no
Have you been in poor health?	yes	no	Did you have skin allergies?	yes	no
Have you been feeling exhausted?	yes	no	Have you had hives or rashes?	yes	no

Total "yes" answers: _____

Table 8

Find your Chapter Total for physical symptoms and then see where this total is located among the four Categories of Responses. From the Category into which your Chapter Total fell, find your number of Stress Points. Write your number of Stress Points in the space proved near the end of this chapter, or onto a scratch sheet.

Stress Totals				
Chapter Totals:	**0 - 2**	**3 - 4**	**5 - 6**	**7+**
Category:	**Excellent**	**Good**	**Fair**	**Worrisome**

As outlined above, place a **0, 1, 2,** or **3,** in the space next to **"Physical Symptoms"**
Stress Points below, or on your scratch sheet.

Table 9

"Physical Symptoms" Stress Points _____

Further information

Theorell, T. and Rahe, R.H. Psychosocial factors and myocardial infarction I, An inpatient study in Sweden. *Journal of Psychosomatic Research*, 15:25-31, 1971.

Rahe, R.H. and Lind, E. Psychosocial factors and sudden cardiac death: A pilot study. *Journal of Psychosomatic Research*, 15:19-24, 1971.

Liljefors, I. and Rahe, R.H. An identical twin study of psychosocial factors in coronary heart disease in Sweden. *Psychosomatic Medicine*, 32:523-542, 1970.

Rahe, R.H., Ward, H.W., and Hayes, V. Brief group therapy in myocardial infarction rehabilitation: Three-to-four-year follow-up of a trial. *Psychosomatic Medicine*, 41:1229-1242, 1979.

Chapter 4: Psychological Symptoms

Fourth Stress Indicator

U. S. Navy Stress Studies

Following my Fellowship in Sweden, I returned to active duty in the Navy and was assigned to study stress and illness in several different groups of naval personnel. These groups included Underwater Demolition Team (UDT) trainees, Navy aviators, and enlisted men and officers serving aboard ship during the Vietnam War. I also helped to design a comprehensive physical and psychological examination for Army and Navy Prisoners of War (POWs) that was administered at the Naval Hospital, San Diego when they returned from captivity.

What types of mental illness symptoms generally result from experiencing severe life stress events? *The number one symptom is anxiety*. Anxiety symptoms include fears, sleep disturbances, dreams of traumatic experiences, poor appetite, and, often, the excessive use of alcohol in attempts to block out these symptoms. *The number two symptom is depression*. Depression results from repeated memories and thoughts of one's performance during trauma, grieving for friends who lost their lives, worrying about what the future may hold, impaired memory and concentration and, in the extreme, thoughts and plans of self-harm and even suicide.

You have undoubtedly read about post-traumatic stress disorder, or PTSD. This mental health disorder, frequently resulting from severe life stresses, has been described by different names since recorded military history. From the mid- 1980s has it been referred to as PTSD. However, this disorder is not limited to persons who have experienced war trauma. It is also seen to occur from childhood to old age following traumas such as abuse, rape, criminal actions, earthquakes, and hurricanes.

Stories in the press about persons with PTSD are generally those of individuals with long-term suffering following their traumas. This has led to a belief that PTSD is a severely disruptive, long lasting, even permanently crippling disorder unresponsive to treatment. This belief is a large distortion of the course of recovery for the majority of individuals experiencing trauma. For example, in a large-scale study of over fifty thousand military men and women, 89% to 92% of those completing combat tours in Afghanistan and Iraq did not report the presence of PTSD on their return home. Even the few men and women who did develop PTSD following their combat tours often showed an improved mental status as they recovered over the next two to three years.

There are four critical areas of influence in relation to the development of PTSD following traumatic experiences. Various combinations of these four areas can facilitate or inhibit the development of PTSD.

The first critical area of influence is Risk versus Resilience. Risks include biological and biographical liabilities such as those you read about in the first chapter of this book. Most important among these risks are poor socialization skills, low educational achievement, excessive alcohol and cigarette use, antisocial behaviors, previous psychiatric illness, and very few "successes with challenges" in their early lives. Resilience factors are the opposite of the risks listed above.

The second critical area of influence is the Trauma Severity. It has frequently been believed that experiencing or witnessing very severe trauma leads directly to PTSD for most everyone. In truth, there are many exceptions. These exceptions are found when one considers different combinations of the four critical areas of influence.

The third area of influence is Concomitant Life Stresses that may reduce an individual's stress tolerance at the time of his or her exposure to trauma. Such stresses may include upsetting personal problems, poor physical or psychological health, emergencies of a spouse and/or children at home, legal problems, and financial problems. These stresses create an additional burden of adjustment for a person coping with a trauma.

The fourth area of critical influence that occurs is the Progress toward Recovery an individual has achieved. Was the person psychologically debriefed following the trauma? Did he or she receive good social support from professionals and/or buddies? Once back home, did he or she get back to work? Did the person start to use excessive amounts of alcohol? Did the person isolate him or herself from friends and family and refuse to seek help? Poor progress toward recovery leads to continuing stress symptoms following trauma.

Looking at various combinations of these four critical areas, the most likely combination that leads to PTSD is: high Risk, many Concomitant Life Stresses, moderate to severe Trauma, and little Progress toward Recovery. A second combination: high Risk, many Concomitant Life Stresses, small to moderate Trauma, and little Progress toward Recovery also may lead to PTSD. Severity of Trauma is, not always predictive for PTSD.

A combination of critical areas of high Resilience, such as few to moderate Concomitant Life Stresses, moderate to severe Trauma, and excellent Progress toward Recovery very often results in no PTSD. These individuals seldom seek medical care and their psychiatric symptoms are few. In recovery, they begin to focus on getting back to work, reestablishing supportive family interactions, restricting their alcohol intake, and putting memories of their traumas into "the basement" of their minds.

An additional area of major influence for Progress toward Recovery is stress training. Specifically designed courses for stress training have been carried out for Air Force and Navy aviators determined at risk for being taken captive following a shoot down of their aircraft. This stress training contributed substantially to the adaptation to captivity for prisoners of war (POWs) in Vietnam. You will read more about Navy POWs from the Vietnam War in a later chapter in this book entitled "Responses to Stress."

Complete the BSCI "Psychological Symptoms" Questions

This BSCI chapter on stress and psychological symptoms are an indication of psychological difficulties in general and not to PTSD in particular. There are some important questions concerning the presence or absence of anxiety and depression in your life—the two most common mental health problems of today. One question in the depression section asks about feelings of hopelessness, and a second question asks about having thoughts of suicide. *A "yes" answer to either of these two questions signals an urgent need for an immediate medical/psychological consultation!*

Psychological Symptoms

Indicate whether you have experienced any of the following symptoms <u>over the past year</u>.

Anxiety

Have you been anxious recently?	yes	no
Have stresses "gotten on your nerves"?	yes	no
Were you ever suddenly fearful?	yes	no
Did you have many troubling thoughts?	yes	no
Were you more easily upset than usual?	yes	no
Did you have trouble sleeping?	yes	no

Depression

Have you been feeling sad and alone?	yes	no
Have you been unhappy and joyless?	yes	no
Has your weight changed a lot?	yes	no
Has your sexual interest declined?	yes	no
Did your life look entirely hopeless?	yes	no
Did you ever wish you were dead?	yes	no

Total "yes" answers: _____

Table 10

Stress Totals			
Chapter Totals:	**0**	**1 - 2**	**3 - 4**	**5+**
Category:	**Excellent**	Good	Fair	**Worrisome**

As outlined above, place a **0, 1, 2,** or **3,** in the space next to **"Psychological Symptoms" Stress Points** below, or on your scratch sheet.

Table 11

Review your scores for symptoms of anxiety and/or depression. If you had a *Fair* or *Worrisome* point total, you definitely should consider a mental health consultation and possible therapy! If your symptoms are chiefly the result of experiencing very severe recent life stresses, you might also benefit from medical treatment. Modern medical care can provide you with medications proven to speed your recovery.

Go back to Chapter 2 and review your results for recent life changes in your life. If you had an Excellent or a Good finding for the numbers and intensities of recent life changes, you probably had similar results for mental health symptoms. Few recent life stresses frequently accompany good to excellent physical and mental health. By this time you know that elevated recent life changes, and severe trauma, tend to go hand in hand with Fair to Worrisome illness symptoms.

Determine your Chapter Total for physical symptoms and then see where this total is found among the four Categories of Responses. From the Category into which your Chapter Total fell, find your number of Stress Points. Write your number of Stress Points in the space proved near the end of this chapter, or onto your scratch sheet.

"Psychological Symptoms" Stress Points ___

Further Information

Rahe, R. H. Anxiety and physical illness. *Journal of Clinical Psychiatry*, 49:26-29, 1988.

Rahe, R.H., Karson, S., Howard, N.S., Rubin, R. T., and Poland, R.E. Psychological and physiological assessments on American hostages freed from captivity in Iran. *Psychosomatic Medicine*, 52:1-16, 1990.

Rahe, R.H. Psychosocial stressors and adjustment disorder: van Gogh's life chart illustrates stress and disease. *Journal of Clinical Psychiatry*, 51:13-17, 1990.

Rahe, R.H. Combat stress with comments on post-traumatic stress disorder. Chapter in: J. Yager and R. P. Liberman, (Eds). *Stress in Psychiatry.* Springer Publishing, New York, 1994.

Chapter 5: Behaviors and Emotions

Fifth Stress Indicator

A Generally Unrecognized Source of Stress

You have now seen that stressful life events can exert both precipitating and predisposing influences on a person's susceptibility to illness and that concurrent physical and psychological illnesses often increase the risk for more illnesses. Additionally, there is still another illness risk category of importance that is often unrecognized.

Precipitating recent life stress events as well as physical and psychological illness symptoms tend to come and go. That is, these events and illnesses challenge us for a few years, but without further major life stresses our health tends to return to normal. Non-adaptive behaviors and emotions, however, are usually learned at an early age and stay with us over our lifetime—unless we make concerted efforts to modify them.

Type A Behavior Pattern

The most publicized unhealthy human behavior pattern is the Type A behavior pattern. Individuals who exhibit this pattern of behaviors and emotions show incessant striving for success, are always in a hurry, try to do more and more in less time, have frequent bursts of anger, and strong impatience with delays. Long hours at work also leave little time for family activities. Sir William Osler, one of the first physicians to treat coronary heart disease patients in this country (as it was a rare illness in the early twentieth century) noted several of these behavioral characteristics in his patients with cardiac pain (angina pectoris). In the mid-1930s, Flanders Dunbar, M.D., an early president of the American

Psychosomatic Society, studied a group of coronary heart disease patients and reaffirmed these findings of non-adaptive behaviors and emotions. In the mid-1950s, Meyer Friedman, M.D., and Ray Rosenman, M.D., both cardiologists, published a series of scientific papers concerning these same behaviors and emotions seen in their patients with coronary disease. They originated the label "Type A behavioral pattern."

Following these publications, other physicians and psychologists carried out dozens of studies of Type A behavior, which led to refinements in testing and in the devising of interventions. In my early Navy studies of patients recovering from a heart attack, I discovered that many of these emotions and behaviors could be modified through group feedback. For example, one patient strongly and loudly denied that he was aggressive and impatient. A second patient laughed and said: "You remind me of me before I started this group." (Other group members had pointed out this second patient's previous aggressive and angry behavior.) Another patient, after being alerted by the group about his reported aggressive driving and impatience with slow traffic, told the group toward the end of his six sessions, "I'm now the driver that I used to honk at!"

Friedman and Rosenman also suggested a Type B behavioral pattern, which was essentially the opposite of Type A. Type B patients in their practice were healthier, happier, and often had less severe coronary heart disease.

In the 1970s, research began on behavioral and emotional characteristics frequently seen in patients with cancer (early subjects were women with breast cancer). This behavioral pattern, similar in some ways to Type A, was called Type C. Both Type As and Type Cs tended to obsess about always being on time for an appointment; both types were very hard working and highly responsible. They both tended to lead very independent lives.

Other aspects of Type C, however, are very different from Type A. Type C individuals show a strong suppression of their emotions, especially anger. Type C people tend to be quiet and courteous, frequently helping others but rarely, if ever, asking for help in return. With their suppression of negative emotions, Type C patients were usually seen as pleasant and cheerful, typically avoiding conflicts, never retaliating if treated badly, and often helpful to others (though seldom pursuing their own desires). Intervention studies for Type C behavior have been carried out. Assertiveness training has been reported to lead to improved health and better rates of survival for cancer patients.

Type C has also been shown to be associated with suppression of immune function in patients with AIDS. A recent report from a large medical center specializing in the treatment AIDS stated that modification of Type C behavior in AIDS patients, using group based assertiveness training, tended to slow the progression of the disease and in some patients even led to improved survival.

Type A behavioral pattern is also associated with elevated blood pressure, high serum cholesterol levels, and increased stomach gastric acid secretion that can lead to peptic ulcer. So like Type C, these behaviors and emotions are not specific for heart disease and cancer, but can also be associated with other illnesses.

Now that there is a Type A, a Type B, and a Type C behavior and emotions pattern, what's next? Very recent studies of patients with coronary heart disease who also suffer from psychological depression, and who typically isolate themselves from others, have been labeled "Type D."

Old Brain and New Brain Behaviors and Emotions

Paul McLean, M.D., a famous neurologist, has examined and described the human brain's oldest to newest regions of development. In the core of our brain is our oldest brain region, which he labeled the "reptilian brain"—as this brain region also is found in reptiles. Next, human beings and other mammals have a more newly developed brain region that surrounds the reptilian brain and specializes in functions concerned with early forms of communication and group living, which he labeled our "old brain," or the "limbic system." Surrounding these two central regions of the brain are two large cerebral hemispheres that control, among other functions, movement, sight, hearing, and communications with the two older central regions. McLean labeled these hemispheres our "new brain." The new brain is functionally divided into several lobes, with the frontal lobe located just behind the forehead. The frontal lobe is a critical region of the new brain devoted to processing our thoughts and behaviors required for successfully living in modern civilization.

Behaviors and emotions coming from our reptilian brain have to do with self-preservation. Two emotions are found there: fear and rage. Fear helps us find and maintain safety when at risk for attack. Rage prepares us for aggressive fighting when needed. Behaviors derived from the reptilian brain include territoriality, selecting leaders, following precedents, deception, and seeking home sites. Taken together, these behaviors and emotions bring to mind the procedures and expectations of the military! Soldiers, in order to survive in battle, must live in their reptilian brains. That is, they often fight for territory, select campsites, follow presidents, use deception when helpful, and employ both stealth and aggression when needed. It is returning to the demands of living in civilization after surviving for months to years living by the reptilian brain that presents some of the biggest challenges of recovery of soldiers returning home!

The limbic system supports more sophisticated behaviors and emotions, which extends the preservation-of-self behaviors of the reptilian brain to emotions and behaviors important in the preservation of the group. The beginnings of speech are found here. Altruism, an emotion that leads an individual to choose to sacrifice his or her life in order to promote preservation of the group, is present in the limbic system as well. Therefore, modern day soldiers also use their limbic systems as they fight for survival of their buddies in their platoon.

The inferior portion of our frontal lobe has extremely important inhibitory pathways directed to the limbic system and the reptilian brain. These inhibitory influences allowed humans to move from living in small groups constantly at war with one another, to adjusting peaceably to life in towns and cities. Our frontal lobe today is our new brain's center of action helping us to adapt and survive the complex demands of twenty-first century civilization.

An example of this new brain inhibition of our reptilian and limbic brains that I tell most every Iraq and Afghanistan veteran that I treat is driving on the freeway. During their combat tour driving vehicles was inherently dangerous. Other unidentified vehicles were presumed to be enemy armed with explosives. Recent digging alongside the road could signal the position of an explosive device. So back home, when they initially drove again on the freeway, they wanted to quickly get to where they were going and felt strong impatience and frequently aggressive anger with cars that delayed them. They had thoughts of "blowing away" drivers that cut in front of them. This is the limbic system and reptilian brain still being active. Once I explained to them how their new brains would assist them to inhibit these anxieties over freeway driving, and further when they discovered that this was indeed the case, they became more optimistic about their recovery.

Most of us are not soldiers returning from combat tours. Still, our reptilian brains are often active and sometimes get us into trouble. Type A persons show many reptilian brain emotions and behaviors. They struggle to achieve more and more success at work, frequently feeling emotions of fear that they won't succeed and aggression towards their competitors. Most all of us, in fact, show some Type A behaviors when driving on the freeway and another driver cuts us off or makes us slow way down for no apparent good reason. These emotions and behaviors in the extreme typify persons exhibiting "road rage."

Complete the BSCI "Behaviors and Emotions" Questions

Answer the behaviors and emotions questions listed in Table 12 below. As you complete your answers, you may note that questions dealing with work, speed, and outlook include several Type A behaviors and emotions, while questions about lack of assertion, emotional suppression, and social inhibition contain many Type C behaviors and emotions.

Determine your Chapter Total for Behaviors and Emotions and then see where this total is found among the four Categories of Responses in Table 13. From the Category into which your Chapter Total fell, find your number of Stress Points. Write your number of Stress Points in the space proved near the end of this chapter, or onto your scratch sheet.

Behaviors and Emotions

Circle your answers.

Work behaviors

Do you work a lot of overtime?	yes	no
Do you concentrate intensely?	yes	no
Are you unable to delegate tasks to others?	yes	no
Do you always have to do a job "right"?	yes	no

Speed

Do you walk, talk, and/or drive fast?	yes	no
Are you often pressed for time?	yes	no
Are you a very competitive person?	yes	no
Do you get angry in slow traffic?	yes	no

Outlook

Are you rarely happy and content?	yes	no
Do you feel out of control over your life?	yes	no
Do you frequently take risks?	yes	no
Do you frequently feel helpless?	yes	no

Assertion

Is it hard for you to "stand up" for yourself?	yes	no
Are you rarely able to say what you want?	yes	no
Do others tend to take advantage of you?	yes	no
If ridiculed, do you just take it?	yes	no

Emotions

When angry, do you usually "keep it inside"?	yes	no
When unhappy, do you seldom tell anyone?	yes	no
If you become angry, do you feel guilty later?	yes	no
Do you generally hide your emotions?	yes	no

Social

Do you usually avoid conflict with others?	yes	no
Is it hard for you to ask for a favor?	yes	no
Do you put off making difficult decisions?	yes	no
Do you rarely get into arguments?	yes	no

Total "yes" answers:_____

Table 12

	Stress Totals			
Chapter Totals:	**0 - 3**	**4 - 6**	**7 - 8**	**9+**
Category:	**Excellent**	**Good**	**Fair**	**Worrisome**

As in the chapters above, place a **0, 1, 2,** or **3,** in the space next to
"Behaviors and Emotions" Stress Points below, or on your scratch sheet.

Table 13

"Behaviors and Emotions" Stress Points _____

Further Information

Friedman, M and Rosenman, R.H., Association of specific overt behavior pattern with blood and cardiovascular findings. *JAMA,* 169:1286, 1959.

Rosenman, R.H., Rahe, R.H., Borhani, N., and Feinleib, M. Heritability of personality and behavior pattern. *Acta Geneticae Medicae et Gamallologie*, 25:221-224, 1974.

Temoshok, L. and Dreher, H. *The Type C Connection: Behavioral Links to Cancer and Your Health.* Random House, New York, 1992.

MacLean, P.D. *The Triune Brain in Evolution.* Plenum, New York, 1990.

Your Total Stress Score

You have now completed the Five Stress Indicators of the BSCI. Transfer your numbers of Stress Points for each chapter to Table 14 below. Find your Total Stress Score by adding your Stress Points for all five chapters. Write this total in the space below or on your scratch sheet. This total will be called upon later in the book when you reach the chapter entitled "Balance Between Stress and Coping."

"Who You Are" Stress Points ____

"Recent Life Changes" Stress Points ____

"Physical Symptoms" Stress Points ____

"Psychological Symptoms" Stress Points ____

"Behaviors and Emotions" Stress Points ____

_____

Total Stress Score: _____

Table 14

Your Total Stress Score will range from 0 to 15 points. The higher your score the greater are your current life challenges. Without adequate coping, the risk of near-future illness is high for you over the next year.

Chapter 6: Health Habits

First Coping Indicator

Complete the BSCI "Health Habits" Questions

Begin this chapter by first answering the BSCI Health Habits questions listed in Table 12 below. Record your sleep habits, physical activity, dietary practice, alcohol intake, tobacco use (if any), and any medications. These are standard health questions, and who amongst us doesn't know the "correct answers?" For instance, we are all aware that low body fat, good physical fitness, a diet high in vegetables and fruit, alcohol restraint, and no tobacco use can lead to a longer life with fewer illnesses. Despite this knowledge, how many of us regularly practice these health-enhancing habits?

Some of these habits are easier to follow than others. Also, each person has a different set of priorities in life and these can either promote or defeat good health. For example, for a cook or chef to maintain a slim figure may be next to impossible. However, if you coach a sport, running and weight workouts may easily fit into your daily schedule. So don't be discouraged if you have some life styles that resist health improvements. As long as you keep working on those habits that are accessible to your way of life, you are on the right track to improving your health.

As you begin the Coping chapters of this book you will find minor changes in your scoring. In the Stress chapters, the higher your Chapter Totals were, the greater your number of Stress Points. In the Coping chapters, the higher your Chapter Totals are, the greater the number of Coping Points. As with Stress Points, Coping Points for a chapter range from 0 to 3.

Health Habits

Circle your answers, then total the points.

Substance Use

Do you smoke cigarettes?	yes (0)	no (2)
Do you have more than 7 drinks per week?	yes (0)	no (2)
Do you use recreational drugs?	yes (0)	no (2)
Are you concerned about your use of medications?	yes (0)	no (2)

Diet

Do you pay close attention to what and how much you eat?	yes (1)	no (0)
Do you eat your meals in pleasant surroundings?	yes (1)	no (0)
Do you eat your meals slowly and calmly?	yes (1)	no (0)

Exercise

Does your work or homelife require some exercise?	yes (1)	no (0)
Do you exercise moderately and regularly?	yes (1)	no (0)
Do you exercise vigorously and regularly?	yes (2)	no (0)

Pace

Are you in control over the pace of your life?	yes (2)	no (0)
Do you feel that you maintain sufficient reserve energy?	yes (1)	no (0)
Do you get enough sleep?	yes (2)	no (0)

Total: _____

Table 15

Coping Totals

Chapter Totals:	0 - 9	10 - 12	13 - 16	17 - 20
Category:	Worrisome	Fair	Good	Excellent
Coping Points:	Worrisome 0,	Fair 1,	Good 2,	Excellent 3

As in the chapters above, place a **0,1,2,** or **3,** in the space next to your **"Health Habits" Coping Points** at the end of the chapter, or on your scratch sheet.

Table 16

Improve Your Health Habits

One way you can improve four health habits all at the same time is by practicing the single health habit of regular physical activity. If you can manage thirty minutes of running, biking, or swimming, three to four times a week, you could lose body fat, increase your muscle mass, probably cut down or even stop smoking if you are a smoker, and become more health conscious. From these four achievements, you might even shift from a high fat and carbohydrate diet to eating more fruits and vegetables. Five for one!

How about other important health habits? Sleep is extremely important! Do you get enough restful sleep? Experts say our bodies need eight and a half hours of sleep a night. Young adults need more and older adults can get by on less. But the majority of us don't get sufficient restful sleep.

Have you heard of *sleep hygiene*? It pertains to following a thoughtful plan regarding your approach to going to bed. Two prime rules are to not exercise heavily or eat a large meal close to retiring. Instead, exercise and eat (reasonably sized meals) in the late afternoon or early evening. Another suggestion is to begin slowing down your day's activities two to three hours before bedtime. Try going to bed close to the same time each evening. Reading before sleep is fine, but don't go to bed to read. If you do, the bedroom tends to become a reading room rather than a sleeping area. Some other sleep-inducing activities include taking a warm bath or shower before bedtime, for as your body cools it promotes sleep. Also, a very light snack, such as a glass of milk, can help you fall asleep. (Grandmother was right when she insisted on this.)

If sleep medicines are used, avoid ones that are potentially habit-forming and may cause memory problems. Lastly, the "gurus of sleep" say to sleep with your body aligned along the north-south axes of the Earth. It lines you up with the magnetic poles. You may have to shift your bed to another position to achieve this suggestion.

Other health habits that keep our brains working in high gear include reading, playing card games, and doing puzzles. Brain activity is as important as physical activity for maintaining our mental health as we age.

One health habit that many people fail to practice is following a reasonable pace of life. Many of us try to do too much over too brief periods of time. (Remember the Type A behavior pattern.) We don't think of taking breaks while pursuing lengthy tasks. I like to use the example of a mountain climber scaling a peak to emphasize the importance of pace. Successful climbers do not constantly strive towards the mountain's peak as they climb, looking to see if it is becoming closer and closer as they hurry up the grade. They do not rush their pace as they get closer to their destination. Instead, they enjoy the scenery along the way, stop regularly for rest breaks and nutrition, and when they arrive at the mountain peak it almost comes as a surprise! Most important is that the climber with pace saves energy for the trip down! How many times have you read of mountain climbers hurrying to get to the top only to run out of strength and endurance on their way back down? Sadly, too many die from exhaustion in the freezing weather.

Like you did in previous chapters, find your Chapter Total from Table 15 by summing the numbers found next to the items you checked. Then, find the Category of Responses in Table 16 where your Chapter Total is located. Write your number of "Health Habits" Coping Points, from 0 to 3, in the space indicated at the end of the chapter or on your scratch sheet.

"Health Habits" Coping Points _____

Further Information

The Surgeon General's Report on Nutrition and Health. U.S. Government Printing Office, Publication Number 88-50810, Washington D.C., 1988.

Cooper, K. *The Aerobics Program for Total Well Being.* M. Evans & Co., New York, 1982.

Golan, R. *Optimal Wellness*. Bantam, New York, 1995.

Dement, W. *Some Just Watch While Some Must Sleep*. Norton Books, London, 1978.

Chapter 7: Social Support

Second Coping Indicator

As in the "Health Habits" chapter above, begin by completing the social support questions from the BSCI in Table 17 below. These questions were derived from a number of studies regarding this coping indicator, and once completed should give you a quick reading of your use of social support for managing stress.

Obtain your Chapter Total from Table 17 and find the Category of Responses in Table 18 where your total is located. Find your number of Coping Points, from 0 to 3, and write it at the end of the chapter, or on a scratch sheet.

Social Support

Circle your answers, then total the points.

When troubled, 1 keep things to myself.	Rarely (2)	Sometimes (1)	Often (0)
There are several people with whom 1 spend time.	Rarely (0)	Sometimes (1)	Often (2)
1 feel that 1 am on the fringe of my circle of friends.	Rarely (2)	Sometimes (1)	Often (0)
1 have friends who will always support me.	Rarely (0)	Sometimes (1)	Often (2)
1 feel no one exists to whom 1 can tell my private concerns.	Rarely (2)	Sometimes (1)	Often (0)
1 frequently feel lonely.	Rarely (2)	Sometimes (1)	Often (0)
1 participate in several social groups.	Rarely (0)	Sometimes (1)	Often (2)
1 get invited to do interesting things with others.	Rarely (0)	Sometimes (1)	Often (2)

Total: _____

Table 17

	Coping Totals			
Chapter Totals:	**0 - 7**	**8 - 10**	**11 - 13**	**14 - 16**
Category:	**Worrisome**	**Fair**	**Good**	**Excellent**

As in the chapters above, place a **0, 1, 2,** or **3,** in the space next to your **"Social Support" Coping Points** or on your scratch sheet.

Table 18

A Social Support Exercise

As I did in the "Who You Are" chapter, I have presented an exercise that has been very popular with persons who participated in my stress and coping workshops. This exercise illustrates some important differences in support that you receive from casual friendships compared to what you gain from your *best* friends.

Figure 2 below, "Where Is Your Social Support?" has four concentric circles of different sizes, designed by Dr. D.A. Tubesing, to represent your layers of social support. You may not want to mark this book during this exercise. If so, start a new scratch sheet and copy Figure 2 onto it. Choose a scratch sheet large enough so that you can write the first names of as many as ten friends in each of the three outer circles.

The smallest circle in the middle of the figure represents you (write "ME" if you are copying the figure). The next surrounding circle is for your family and close friends. You can also include pets here. The circle outside of the one for family and friends is for your friends at work. Lastly, the outermost circle is for your friends in your community.

You begin this exercise by writing the first names of family members and close friends in their designated circle. Then, do the same for friends that you have at work. Finally, write the first names of friends in your community.

Now, review the all the names you have written down in the three circles and draw a circle around those names with whom you contact regularly – either by talking with them on the phone or by seeing them in person. Ready for the clincher? Go back and review all the names that you have circled, and draw a star next to those who are your *best* friends. A best friend is one whom you would first think to call if you urgently needed help. A best friend would then stop whatever they were doing and come to your aid as quickly as possible! They would not say, "I'm terribly busy right now. Perhaps you should call 911?"

Look at your total number of friends that you listed in all three circles. This number of friendships is called your *social support network*. These networks can be quite large, but a large network may not be all that supportive for you in times of need. So move on from totaling the number of people in your network to counting the names that you placed circles around. Circled names indicate the *utilization of your network*. Friends become closer friends when you keep in touch! In contrast to the size of your network, the greater the number of friends with whom you keep in touch, the higher your potential will be for social support in times of need. Your most supportive friends will be your *best friends* and you placed a star by their names. These persons represent the *depth of your utilization network.* The more stars you drew the greater is this depth.

Individuals facing extremely dangerous life challenges together quickly develop best friends. See chapter titled "Responses to Stress" for examples of this phenomenon. Further information concerning how to "grow" best friends is found in the last chapter, "Purpose and Connection."

Where Is Your Social Support?

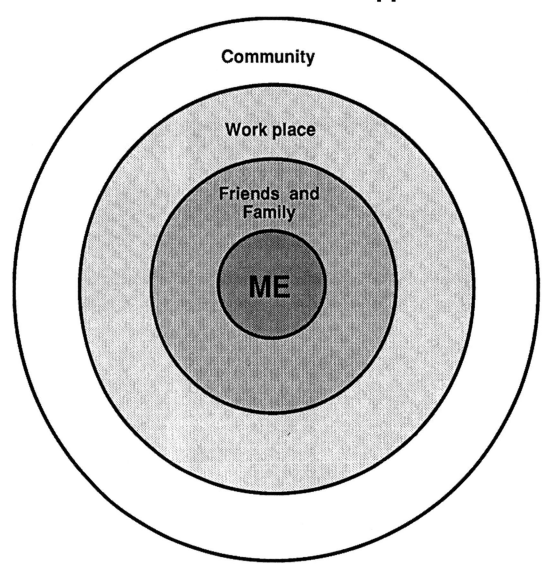

Community

Work place

Friends and Family

ME

Figure 2

"Social Support" Coping Points _____

Further Information

Wolf, S. and Bruhn, J.G. *The Power of Clan: The Influence of Human Relationships on Heart Disease*. Transaction Publishers, New Brunswick, New Jersey, 1993.

Thoits, P.A. Stress, coping, and social support processes. *J. Health and Soc. Behav.,* Extra Issue, 53-79, 1995.

Rahe, R.H., Ward, H.W., and Hayes, V. Brief group therapy in myocardial infarction rehabilitation: Three-to-four-year follow-up of a controlled trial. *Psychosomatic Medicine*, 41:1229-1242, 1979.

Tubesing, D.A. *Structured Exercises in Stress Management.* Whole Person Associates, Inc., Duluth, 1988.

Chapter 8: Responses to Stress

Third Coping Indicator

How we think and act when we face extremely challenging life situations strongly influences our body's responses to this stress! These thoughts and actions can magnify, modify, or even cancel our physical and psychological reactions. Perhaps the most telling examples of both adaptive and non-adaptive reactions to severe stress have come from military history. Let's begin with a description of psychological blindness resulting from frightening combat stress, recorded by Herodotus in The Battle of Marathon, waged in 490 BC:

Epizelus, an Athenian soldier, was fighting bravely when he suddenly lost the sight of both eyes, though nothing had touched him anywhere...he continued blind as long as he lived...he thought he was opposed by a man of great stature in heavy armor, whose beard overshadowed his shield; but the phantom passed him by and killed the man at his side.

Psychological loss of sight resulting from a single episode of overwhelming life stress rarely occurs, but it is still seen today. In contrast, the most common maladaptive response to cumulative wartime stress is psychological depression. Shakespeare gave us an extremely accurate description of this phenomenon in his play *Henry IV*. Lady Percy bemoans the physical and psychological features of Henry's depression below:

Tell me, sweet lord, what is't that takes from thee

Thy stomach, pleasure, and thy golden sleep?

Why dost thou bend thine eyes upon the earth,

And start so often when thou sit'st alone?

Why has thou lost the fresh blood in thy cheeks,

and given my treasures and my rights of thee

To thick-eyed musing and cursed melancholy?

In thy faint slumbers I by thee have watch'd,

And heard thee murmur tales of iron wars.

Many American soldiers, from the Civil War to modern day military actions in Afghanistan and Iraq, have developed cardiac (Irritable Heart), brain (Shell Shock, Traumatic Brain Injury), and psychological illnesses (Battle Neurosis, Combat Stress, Post Traumatic Stress Disorder) attributable to their psychological and physical reactions to the stresses of war. Thankfully, these soldiers are in the minority of all men and women sent in harm's way. The question arises: "How do these soldiers, exposed to similar brutal wartime stresses, escape from developing these disorders?"

Successful Adaptation to Long-Term Military Stress

It is a rare opportunity to obtain long-term physical and psychological information on a group of military men who endured and survived years of one of the most stressful experiences of wartime—being captured and held as prisoners-of-war (POW). This information was obtained for 133 Navy aviators held in captivity from 1 to 8 years before their release in 1973. The experiences of these men were gathered and analyzed by research personnel in my command at the Naval Health Research Center, San Diego, California. In the early 1980s, I collected similar physical and psychological information from over half of the fifty-two military and civilian hostages held captive at the U.S. Embassy in Iran for 444 days.

Both groups displayed similarities in those psychological and physical stresses received from their captors. Physical torture, mock executions, and solitary confinement, especially that experienced by the POWs, were grueling. During their first months of captivity, many experienced psychological depression. Prolonged physical and social deprivations, along with indefinite terms of confinement, weighed heavily. As medical officers in the United States preparing to receive these men (along with two women who were also held in Iran), we were extremely worried about a possible legacy of severe and lasting illnesses.

For the captives, however, adaptive thoughts and behaviors began to develop very early in captivity. One returned POW, Lieutenant Commander John McGrath, who was held prisoner for six years, published a small volume of sketches depicting both stresses and coping with captivity after his release. Three of his sketches are presented in this chapter (Figures 3, 4, 6).

Some of the most difficult stresses that POWs endured were daily physical beatings, being tightly roped and/or chained while in their cells, having rats crawl over them during night, and surviving on minimal food. During their first years at the "Hanoi Hilton," as they called their prison, they were also forbidden to see or speak to another POW. They were taken to the latrine and to interrogations one prisoner at a time.

Interrogations were particularly challenging for the POWs. The men were asked repeatedly to reveal U.S. Navy military information despite guidelines set forth in the Geneva Convention stating that captured enemy combatants only need to give their name, rank, and service number. When the POWs refused to cooperate with interrogators, they were cruelly beaten, forced to walk on their knees over pieces of broken glass, had rifles put to their heads and triggers pulled in mock executions, and they were often tied so tightly in ropes and/or chains that their shoulders would dislocate.

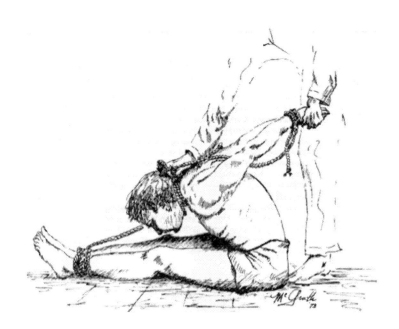

Figure 3

The captives soon realized that if they did not give a little information to their interrogators, they would eventually die from the especially brutal torture that was administered to total resistors. So each man soon learned just how much torture he could endure before having to give some information to his interrogator. Information that they gave was usually non-critical military operations, and even that was often cleverly fabricated. The POW could then rest and partially recover from his beatings for a day or two before his interrogator would discover the lies and bring him back for further torture and interrogation.

Aside from personal torture, POWs frequently stated that a more severe stress was hearing other POWs being tortured! Additionally, many said that the most difficult stress of all was isolation. Thus, an extremely powerful coping strategy used during the first years of captivity was to break this isolation by secretly placing notes where other POWs might find them, such as behind the toilet in the latrine, and using the tap code.

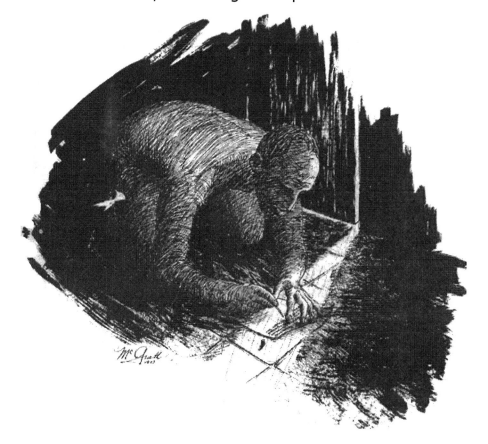

Figure 4

The tap code requires establishing a mental picture of the English alphabet as five rows of five letters aligned with the first row on top, the second row underneath the first, and so on with the fifth row on the bottom. This arrangement also made for five columns of letters going from left to right, with each column comprised of five letters. As there are twenty-six letters in the English alphabet, one letter has to be "discarded." The discarded letter was "k." If a "k" was needed in a word the letter "c" was substituted, as "c" often has a "k" sound in words such as "can." See Figure 5 below for this arrangement of letters.

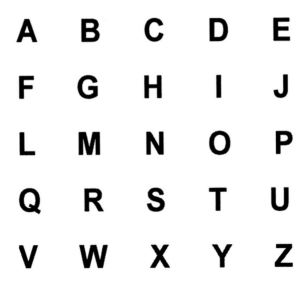

Figure 5

Keeping this picture in mind, two sets of taps were used to identify a letter. The first tapping, from one to five taps, indicated the row that contained the letter being communicated. For example, one tap would indicate the top row, two taps the second row, and on up to five taps signaling the bottom row. The second set of taps, from one to five, indicated the column of letters containing the communicated letter. The first column of letters on the left side of the schema is indicated by one tap. The next column to the right was identified by two taps, and so forth on to the fifth column to the right (five taps).

As the men initially did not have materials, such as charcoal and paper, to write the scheme down, they learned to use a mental picture of the display (Figure 5). Try testing yourself by not looking at Figure 5 and see if you can identify the following word? tap tap... tap tap tap, tap...tap tap tap tap tap, tap tap tap...tap, tap tap tap... tap, tap tap tap...tap tap tap tap. (Did you peak at Figure 5?)

You may think it would take a very long time to spell out a sentence or two. That would be the case as a man first learned the code. However, the men soon began creating abbreviations for commonly used words. Some words were abbreviated to just their first letter. After a torture session when the POW was being taken back to his cell, POWs nearby would tap "GBU," the first letters for the words "God bless you."

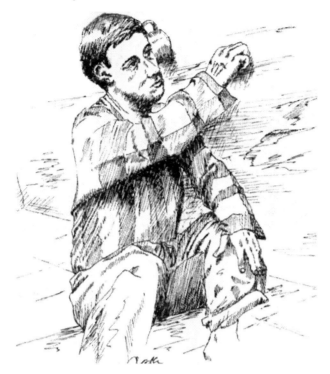

Figure 6

Over their final years in captivity, the men were allowed to spend increasing amounts of time together in a single large room. Here, the social support derived from other captives became enormous. A man would propose to share a skill, or an interest, that he had with others who might be interested. For instance, a person who knew French would offer to start a French class. Others taught their hobbies. Group singing, and singing as loud as they could, provided enormous support. A non-denominational church service was held every Sunday.

The immense bonding between most of the POWs, as well as their respect for following military procedures, resulted in an orderly and highly emotional time when their release was politically achieved. Senator John McCain, who was held as one of the POWs for over five years, illustrated this group bond. As his father was a full admiral on active duty in the Navy while McCain was held captive, the powers in Hanoi offered him an early release. He refused, saying that he would only leave prison when all the other POWs were released- and in the order of their dates of captivity.

Initial and Follow-up Physical and Psychological Exams

What we found upon the return of these two groups of men for yearly follow-up was astoundingly positive! For the Navy returned POWs, their first-year examinations revealed that nearly 70% were both physically and mentally healthy! Moreover, these initially healthy men remained in excellent to good health over the next five years of U.S. Navy funded follow up. (Those with good rather than excellent health reported predominantly minor problems.) The other 30% of the POW group were found to have one or more major illnesses during their first-year exams and continued to report lingering illnesses across the next five years.

The Iranian hostage group showed very similar results over two years of U. S. Government funded follow-up, in that 70% of the former hostages were found to be in excellent to good health on their initial physical and psychological exams. Two of three initially healthy former hostages remained in excellent to good heath by the end of the second follow-up year. (Those with good rather than excellent health reported predominantly minor illnesses over these two years.) For the 30% of former hostages with one or more significant illnesses discovered on their initial exam, seven out of ten remained in ill health at the end of their second follow-up year. Of the continuing illnesses reported in this second group, 60% were major in severity.

What Does This POW and Hostage Data Mean for Us?

These studies found that persons who coped well with their significant stresses of captivity developed few physical and psychological problems during captivity, on their initial exams, and over follow-up. In contrast, those who reported several difficulties during captivity frequently continued to experience physical and psychological problems upon release and over follow-up. Note here the long term health significance of success with challenges during captivity?

Persons successfully adapting to the stresses of captivity frequently had plentiful biological and biographical assets—as you read about in the "Who You Are" chapter. During their challenging stresses, they frequently remembered, and put into practice, prior stress training. High intelligence also led to coming up with clever ways to deal with the stresses. Ability to use social support was highly characteristic for the successful responders. *What you have learned from this chapter should now help you to more successfully manage future life stresses that may arise in your life!*

Posttraumatic Growth

Before leaving this topic, mention should be made of a life-enhancing maturation that survivors of stressful life situations often experience. This maturation is called "posttraumatic growth" and it is characterized by an increased appreciation for life, creating more meaningful personal relationships, a sense of personal strength, a more fulfilling set of life priorities, and, often, a richer existential and spiritual life. A new respect for the sacrifices of parents, siblings, and others is also reported. I frequently said to survivors of severe stress situations: "I know you didn't volunteer for this experience, but after having successfully survived it, do you see yourself as a better person in some ways?" I frequently obtained responses that were extremely similar to the examples given above.

Complete the BSCI "Responses to Stress" Questions

As you answer these questions regarding your responses to stress, you will find some questions that are positive responses to stress while others are negative ones. These questions came from the extensive research in coping with stress by Richard Lazarus, PhD, and Susan Folkman, PhD, at the University of California, San Francisco. I have given these questions to hundreds of very successful men and women and have been astonished to see how few positive responses and how many negative ones that these successful men and women report. Despite their achievements on the job, they still showed room for growth!

Responses to Stress

Circle your answers, then total the points for each of the sections below.

Blame myself for my problems.	Rarely (2)	Sometimes (1)	Often (0)
Focus on something good that will come from situations.	Rarely (0)	Sometimes (1)	Often (2)
Wish the situation would go away.	Rarely (2)	Sometimes (1)	Often (0)
Try to forget the whole thing.	Rarely (2)	Sometimes (1)	Often (0)
Make a plan for action.	Rarely (0)	Sometimes (1)	Often (2)
Change or grow as a person in a good way.	Rarely (0)	Sometimes (1)	Often (2)
Criticize or lecture myself.	Rarely (2)	Sometimes (1)	Often (0)
Ignore the problem.	Rarely (2)	Sometimes (1)	Often (0)
Ask someone 1 respect for advice.	Rarely (0)	Sometimes (1)	Often (2)
Wish that 1 could change how 1 feel.	Rarely (2)	Sometimes (1)	Often (0)

Total: _____

Table 19

How did you do on these questions? Did you subscribe to some of the unhelpful responses? If so, you may have discovered some need for improvement in these areas! Many of these improvements require an "undo it yourself" approach.

Coping Totals

Chapter Totals:	0 - 9	10 - 12	13 - 16	17 - 20
Category:	Worrisome	Fair	Good	Excellent

As in the chapters above, place a **0, 1, 2,** or **3,** in the space next to your **"Reactions to Stress" Coping Points** or on your scratch sheet.

Table 20

Obtain your Chapter Total from Table 19 and find the Category of Responses in Table 20 where your total is located. Find your number of Coping Points and write this number in the space below, or on your scratch sheet.

"Responses to Stress" Coping Points _____

Further Information

McGrath, J. *PRISONER OF WAR. Six Years in Hanoi.* Naval Institute Press, 1975.

Hubbell, J. *POW: A Definitive History of the American Prisoner-of-War Experience in Vietnam, 1964-1973*. Readers Digest Press, New York, 1978.

Segal, J., Jones, D.R., and Rahe, R.H. Recommendations for future P.O.W. activities. In: *Proceedings of the Veterans Administration Conference of Vietnam Prisoners of War.* U.S. Government Printing Office, 1987.

Folkman, S. and Lazarus, R. An analysis of coping in a middle-aged community sample. *J. Health Soc. Behav.*, 21:219-239,1980.

Richlin, M., Shale, J.H., and Rahe, R.H. Five-year medical follow-up of Navy POW's repatriated from Vietnam: Preliminary results. *U.S. Navy Medicine*, 71:19-26, 1980.

Rahe, R.H. Life change, stress responsively, and captivity research. *Psychosomatic Medicine*, 52:373-396, 1990.

Rahe, R.H. Adaptation to captivity. Chapter in: G. Fink (Ed). *Encyclopedia of Stress* (Revised). Elsevier, pp 388-391, 2007.

Rahe, R.H. Recovery from captivity. Chapter in: G. Fink (Ed). *Encyclopedia of Stress* (Revised). Elsevier, pp 392-396, 2007

Chapter 9: Life Satisfactions

Fourth Coping Indicator

What Gets You Out of Bed in the Mornings?

For some people, it's looking forward to spending time with their children. For others, it is their love of work. Still others might say it's taking walks in Nature. I know a surgeon who is close to sixty years old who told me recently, "It's wind surfing!" Life satisfactions bring joy into our lives, and we tend to thrive, both psychologically and physically, from these activities.

High satisfaction in one area of your life can also balance a lack of satisfaction in another. For example, persons with jobs that give them little joy and pleasure may find that a warm and supportive family life balances things out. What you want to avoid is a life of Sisyphus. Sisyphus, a legendary king in Greece, was punished for his cruel deeds during his lifetime by being sentenced, for eternity, to push a large and heavy stone up a tall hill and place it at the top. But as the top of the hill was pointed, when Sisyphus pushed the stone the top it rolled down the other side. His afterlife was, therefore, one of endless joyless striving.

Is your life one of joyless striving? If so, it can lead to high blood pressure, elevated blood fats, poor control of body sugar, thyroid disease, and a host of other illnesses. Perhaps it's time for some immediate modifications, leading to increased life satisfactions.

Complete the BSCI "Life Satisfactions" Questions

Current Life Satisfactions

Pleased with my state of health.	Rarely (0)	Sometimes (1)	Often (2)
Unhappy with my work situation.	Rarely (2)	Sometimes (1)	Often (0)
Happy with my level of job security.	Rarely (0)	Sometimes (1)	Often (2)
Dissatisfied with my boss(es).	Rarely (2)	Sometimes (1)	Often (0)
Satisfied with my personal relationships.	Rarely (0)	Sometimes (1)	Often (2)
Concerned with family problems.	Rarely (2)	Sometimes (1)	Often (0)
Satisfied with my financial situation.	Rarely (0)	Sometimes (1)	Often (2)
Dissatisfied with my current housing or neighborhood.	Rarely (2)	Sometimes (1)	Often (0)

Total: _____

Table 21

Coping Totals

Chapter Totals:	0 - 7	8 - 10	11 - 13	14 - 16
Category:	Worrisome	Fair	Good	Excellent

As in the chapters above, place a **0, 1, 2,** or **3,** in the space next to your **"Life Satisfactions" Coping Points** or on your scratch sheet.

Table 22

Obtain your Chapter Total from Table 21 and find the Category of Responses in Table 22 where your total is located. Find your number of Coping Points and write this number in the space placed at the end of this chapter, or on your scratch sheet.

Additional Pathways to Life Satisfactions

When I was leading my stress and coping workshops in the U.S., Europe, Brazil, and Australia, I was frequently asked: "I know I need more satisfactions in my life, but how can I find them?" So in writing this book I have selected four of my suggestions that I had provided to theses attendees. See if they give you a push.

Humanize your work

A story is told of three stonecutters in Ancient Egypt who toiled daily shaping stones from large pieces of granite that were to be used to build the pyramids. One day, the first worker said in disgust that he hated this job because every day he had to do the same heavy work over and over. The second worker, in a happier voice, said that although it was very repetitive and laborious work he was content because the money he made paid for a home, food, and clothing for his family. The third worker turned to the other two and also agreed that the work was both laborious and tedious, but he was proud to be crafting the stones to be used to build the Pharaoh's glorious pyramids that would remain standing for centuries and bring lasting fame to Egypt.

Can you see how the second and third worker humanized their job? From these examples you might find that though your views of your job won't change the work itself, they can change how you evaluate your work. Does your job enrich your community, and possibly your society?

An interest in the arts

Another area of life satisfaction that many people enjoy is an interest in the arts. If you presently don't take time to enjoy music, literature, the theater, opera, photography, or other areas of artistic expression, this could be a new area of satisfaction for you. There are several different types of music, paintings, sculpture, and ceramics on display in most art museums; but in order to fully enjoy an area in the arts you may find it helpful to first do some basic study.

Books on the history of the area of the arts you choose to pursue are a good place to start. With some knowledge derived from books, you can move on to museums, or attend a concert, knowing a bit more what to expect. Pick a museum or a theater in the city where you live, or a nearby city if you live in a small town. You'll know when you've picked a satisfying new interest when you begin planning trips to visit larger libraries, more comprehensive museums, or even highly celebrated performances in cities farther and farther from your home!

Once you have developed a new and enjoyable interest in the arts, you will likely feel more in touch with the lives of the men and women whose works inspire you. You might also even discover study groups where you can meet new and knowledgeable persons who can help further expand your horizons. Perhaps these new interests will even stimulate members of your family to join you on your new path.

Enjoyable physical activity

Let's face it. Regular physical activity can be a drag! But you know how healthful physical activity can nourish your heart, lungs, muscles, and trim body weight. Many people decide on jogging for their first choice of exercise, but often their bodies were not designed for running. Don't be discouraged of you don't do well with jogging as there are other avenues of exercise available.

The key to picking and maintaining regular physical fitness is to choose an activity that you find enjoyable! If you have bad knees, consider swimming. Swimming is nearly "anti-gravity," as the water supports a good part of your body weight. Most new swimmers find they initially don't like the smell of chlorinated swimming pool water, but this early dislike generally fades away the more often they come to the pool.

Another enjoyable regular exercise is walking. Walking in parks, in wooded areas, or even through beautiful neighborhoods are good places to begin. Find locations that are restful and not crowded. Walk slowly at first for no more than half a mile or so. Soon, your pace and distance will start to increase and you'll even begin to burn some calories. You might next try some brisk walking on flat stretches.

The key to maintaining enjoyable physical activity is to do it with a buddy! Pick someone with whom you already enjoy talking, as there will be plenty of time for conversation. On days when you don't feel like walking, swimming, jogging, etc., you will do it anyway because you'll know that your buddy will be there waiting for you—and vice versa. After the exercise, you and your buddy (or perhaps several buddies by this time) may possibly begin rewarding yourselves with a visit to a coffee shop and having an occasional, well-deserved, healthy cookie.

Create healthy, artful dining

When I conducted workshops for stressed executives, I routinely asked them what they ate for breakfast. I was confronted over and over by how poorly these successful, intelligent men and women eat! The usual response I received was: "Coffee (often several cups) and a sweet roll." No juice, no cereals, no eggs, no nourishment! If a sweet roll is hard on your body's sugar balance, adding caffeine from coffee or tea increases your sugar level even higher! This "diet" provides a short burst of energy that lasts about thirty to forty minutes. To make matters worse, most of my workshop executives ate this "meal" on the run.

I won't even begin to mention their "power lunches" and high calorie dinners. These executives frequently said they didn't have the time or interest to eat well. Their priorities were work (though often not humanized), fighting traffic, frequent consumption of alcohol, watching TV, and sleep (usually not enough).

Creating healthy meals takes knowledge, careful shopping, and planning. A healthy diet can be promoted through artful dining. Have your breakfast in a cozy and well-lit area. Use tasteful dishware and cutlery. A healthy breakfast can also be quick. A cup of yogurt, fruit juice, toast with peanut butter, and one cup of coffee can be consumed leisurely in five to ten minutes. For children, yogurt, fruit, vitamin powder, and milk can be combined in a blender and served to them in their favorite mug, to be consumed as they are being driven to the school bus.

A healthy lunch is more difficult to orchestrate. I still use a lunchbox to carry my healthy (meat and cheese, not peanut butter and jelly) sandwiches and fruit. I do add a (not always healthy) cookie or two. Then, I pick a quiet time and restful place to eat. I don't take a lunch hour, or even half-hour, but I eat slowly. I avoid eating in crowded cafeterias.

Dinner can be a masterpiece. We now know that a glass or two of wine with dinner is good for our hearts as well as for relaxation. Planning dinners for the week and doing the necessary shopping is best accomplished the prior weekend. Use a dining area that is separate from your breakfast nook. Artfully arranging the dishes makes your food more inviting. Finding fresh fish, when available, is an easy way to prepare a healthy and artful dinner. Meat and potatoes are not necessarily bad for you if eaten in reasonable quantities. Restaurants in the United States serve far too much food on your plate, so choose your dining out establishments with your health in mind!

"Life Satisfactions" Coping Points _____

Further Information

Antonovsky, A. *Health, Stress, and Coping*. Jossey-Bass, San Francisco, 1979.

Kabat-Zinn, J. *Wherever You Go, There You Are*. Hyperion, New York, 1994.

Martin, F. D. and Jacobus, L.A. *The Humanities Through the Arts*. McGraw-Hill, New York, 2003.

Kamien, R. *Music, an Appreciation, Brief*. Hebrew University Press, Jerusalem, 2008.

Chapter 10: Purpose and Connections

Fifth Coping Indicator

What Makes Your Life Worth Living?

Try to define the chief purposes of your life. Are your activities, including your work, helpful to others, to society, to the earth? What important beliefs and life directions exist for you? This chapter explores purposes in your life along with your connections with others, and even the earth.

The questions you are to answer below about purpose and connection in your life were recently translated into Hungarian and given to several hundred citizens of the nation's capital city of Budapest. Those who answered that they had important purpose and connections in their lives were found to be twice as healthy as those others without these life dimensions. In a country that has recently shifted from communism to democracy, resulting in many life changes and stresses for inhabitants, having purpose and connection in their lives appeared to protect many citizens from Hungary's recently experienced their country's very large increase in coronary heart disease.

Complete the BSCI "Purpose and Connection" Questions

Complete the BSCI Purpose and Connection questions. Sum your Chapter Total from the questions in Table 23 below. Find the Category of Responses that contains your number of Coping Points from Table 24, and place this number in the space at the end of this chapter or on your scratch sheet.

Purpose and Connection

1 feel my life is part of some larger plan.	Rarely (0)	Sometimes (1)	Often (2)
My life has no direction and meaning.	Rarely (2)	Sometimes (1)	Often (0)
Many things in life give me great joy.	Rarely (0)	Sometimes (1)	Often (2)
1 am able to forgive myself and others.	Rarely (0)	Sometimes (1)	Often (2)
1 doubt that my life makes a difference.	Rarely (2)	Sometimes (1)	Often (0)
My values and beliefs guide me daily.	Rarely (0)	Sometimes (1)	Often (2)
1 feel in tune with people around me.	Rarely (0)	Sometimes (1)	Often (2)
1 am at peace with my place in life.	Rarely (0)	Sometimes (1)	Often (2)

Total: _____

Table 23

Coping Totals

Chapter Totals:	0 - 7	8 - 10	11 - 13	14 - 16
Category:	Worrisome	Fair	Good	Excellent

As in the chapters above, place a **0, 1, 2,** or **3,** in the space next to your **"Purpose and Connection" Coping Points** or on your scratch sheet.

Table 24

How did you do on the Purpose and Connections questions? Did you land in the Good or Excellent category? If so, you have a powerful area of coping in your life. Were you in the Fair or Worrisome category? As in the Life Satisfactions chapter, I have added some Additional Pathways to Purpose and Connection that may lead you to increasing this coping area for good results.

Additional Pathways to Purpose and Connection

Join a community project

Few activities in life give us back the positive returns we receive when helping others less fortunate than ourselves! These returns are even greater when we help those persons living in our own community. In this era of crowded towns and cities, there is a lack of feeling that we are part of the community that surrounds us. Yet, if you look, you probably will find many community services agencies near where you live that would greatly appreciate help from volunteers.

Schools and libraries are often searching to find mentors for children who are having trouble with reading, mathematics, and so forth. Blood banks need for volunteers to help calm donors and make sure they eat and drink something before leaving the clinic after donating a pint of blood. Driving elderly citizens who live alone to their medical appointments and taking them back home again afterwards is another wonderful opportunity for community service. Joining a service organization is a sure-fire way of participating in opportunities to aid community projects. Look around and you'll find something!

Become a true neighbor

One community to which we all belong is the neighborhood in which we live. We may have lived there for several years and never learned the names of our closest neighbors—much less anything more personal about them.

Here's a tried and true way to break down such a barrier. Bake or buy some cookies, and bring a plate of these goodies with you as you knock on the door of a close neighbor's home early one evening. An introduction might go something like this: "I've seen you frequently in your yard, walking your dog, when I'm driving in and out of my garage, and so on, but I'm ashamed to say that I've never stopped to get to know you. I'm _____, and this is my husband /wife/ partner, _____, and these are some of our favorite cookies."

During your first brief talk together, you might bring up what you like about the neighborhood and learn their likes and dislikes. Ask them if they know their neighbors well and compliment them if they do. You may even learn of nearby couples and families with similar occupations and activities as yours.

A next step would be to plan a simple barbeque, or wine and cheese snack, with your new neighborhood friends, and ask them to invite one or two other neighbors who also live near you. During this get-together, you might inquire about any existing community projects, such as making the neighborhood more beautiful or a safer place to live. This could lead to a small beautification project or the beginning of a crime prevention program with help from local police.

Such programs could begin to interest even more neighbors to become involved, and before you know it, you have started your own little community. You now wave to one another as you drive by, keep an eye on each other's house when on travel, and find that you are truly enjoying living in your home-grown community.

Grow additional best friends

In line with what you've just read above about becoming a true neighbor, very similar steps can be taken to develop new best friends. I like the concept of "growing" a best friend because growing is a slow process that takes lots of nourishment. We are focusing now on developing new best friends and not just making new acquaintances.

As you may remember from Chapter 6, "Social Support: the Second Coping Indicator," a best friend is one who, if you called and said that you needed immediate help, would drop whatever they were doing and come over to assist you. When you completed the Social Support Exercise, do you remember how many best friends you had? In my experience leading stress workshops, I have found that it is rare if a person can list more than three or four such friends. Some can't list even one person. This is an area frequently needing attention!

To begin the growth of a new best friend, use your intuition to discover with whom among your current acquaintances you felt an immediate kinship on your first or second meeting. Kinship means that you felt quite comfortable talking with this person and even quickly discovered some mutual experiences and interests. Then, as in the above section of becoming a true neighbor, set up a casual meeting for coffee or lunch. Once you and your friend start sharing stories about life, society, the economy, and so on, you both will know if a deeper friendship is possible. If so, begin fertilizing the friendship with telephone calls and further get-togethers! You have begun the growth of a new best friend.

Find wisdom and humor in life (it's often lurking in the strangest places)

After having lived several decades of life, I was struck by a realization that certain "truths" of life are becoming evident. Many of my early idealistic notions about my occupation and society have proven to be wishful thinking. Selected observations of human behavior, when seen over and over again, began to represent truths to me. For example, working as I have done with social service organizations designed to aid persons displaced by disasters eventually altered my earlier beliefs of their totally selfless service.

Many examples of truths in life are found in the wisdom-imbedded humor of authors such as Mark Twain. Humor also helps lessen life disappointments. One Navy POW overheard a newly captured aviator talking to himself after being thrown into a neighboring prison cell: "My recruiter said joining the Navy would be an adventure, but he didn't mention anything about this!" The POW overhearing this lament said that he laughed long and hard from sharing the humor in this statement.

Life truths also come from reading books written by knowledgeable authors. You can't read Thomas Mann's *Magic Mountain* without obtaining a personal and emotional understanding of the lives led by tuberculosis patients confined for endless years to a sanitarium. Aleksandr Solzhenitsyn's prizewinning novel *One Day in the Life of Ivan Denisovich* leaves you with a disturbingly accurate understanding of the cruel an inhumane treatment of political prisoners in Stalinist Russia.

Increase spirituality in your life

Religion can certainly be an important part of spirituality, but the field of spirituality is larger than a single religion. Some health practices, such as meditation, often have a spiritual basis. Beliefs in our close relationships with animals, trees, even mountains and rivers, make up central features of many Native Americans' spirituality. By and large, these spiritual areas in life lead to feelings of belonging and responsibility.

A Vietnam War veteran who impressed me greatly from his work leading to his recovery from severe PTSD said that the most helpful step he took was developing a meditation practice. He found that until he could clear his mind from repeatedly focusing on past traumas and recriminations, could he experience peace. When he began leading a life centered on helping others rather than remembering his past, he became physically and mentally strong. He has literally walked across the United States three times, sharing his spirituality with those he meets along the way.

The Dalai Lama sends out yearly advice, and one piece of advice he sent this year is: "Spend some time alone every day." In this age of cellular phones, crowded cities, radio and television, it is extremely difficult to be alone without making a time and place for it. Once alone, listen and enjoy the silence! Find a spot in nature to admire its beauty. Breathe fully, and let your tensions release!

"Purpose and Connection" Coping Points _____

Further Information

Skrabski, A., Kopp, M., Sandor, R., Janos, R., and Rahe, R.H. Life mMeaning: An iImportant dDeterminant of pPerceived hHealth in the Hungarian pPopulation. *International Journal of Behavioral Medicine*, 12: 76-82, 2005.

Dossey, L. *Healing Words: The Power of Prayer and the Practice of Medicine.* Harper, San Francisco, 1993.

Debats, D. L. *Meaning in Life: Clinical Relevance and Predictive Power. British J. Clin. Psychol.,* 35:503-516,1996.

Remen, R. N. *Kitchen Table Wisdom: Stories That Heal*. The Berkley Publishing Group, New York, 1996.

Your Total Coping Score

You have now completed the five Coping Indicators. Transfer your numbers of chapter Coping Points from each chapter to Table 11 below. Determine your Total Coping Score by adding all your Coping Points from the five chapters.

"Health Habits" Coping Points _____

"Social Support" Coping Points _____

"Responses to Stress" Coping Points _____

"Life Satisfactions" Coping Points _____

"Purpose and Connection" Coping Points _____

_____

Total Coping Score: _____

Table 25

Your Total Coping Score will range from 0 to 15. The higher your score, the greater your coping skills for handling life challenge. With adequate coping your risk for illness over the next year is reduced. You will learn more about your Stress and Coping Balance, and its measures for resilience, in the next chapter.

Chapter 11: Balance Between Stress and Coping

You are now ready to compare your Total Stress Score to your Total Coping Score on the Stress and Coping Relationship Graph, presented in Figure 7. This graph plots Stress Totals, from 0 to 15 points, on the vertical axis and plots Coping Totals, from 0 to 15 points, along the horizontal axis. To find your Stress and Coping Balance, put your finger at the bottom of the vertical axis, and move it up until you come to your Total Stress Score. Make a light pencil mark at that place along this axis. Next, put your finger back to where you started, and move it along the horizontal axis until you come to your Total Coping Score. Mark that spot lightly. Now, putting your left index finger on the mark you made for your Total Stress Score and your right index finger on your mark you made for your Total Coping Score, move your left finger straight across the graph and your right finger straight up the graph until they meet. Lightly draw a star at this intersection of your two total scores.

In what section of the graph is your star located? If it is in the **Balance** section, then your risk for near-future illness is moderately low. Your total coping equals, or nearly equals, your total stress. Your only worry here is that if new stresses suddenly occur in your life, your star will move up into **Illness Risk** categories. For this reason, I always suggest to persons in the **Balance** section of the graph to work on building a little more coping as a cushion. If they build more coping and no new stresses occur, their star might move down into the **Wellness** categories of the graph.

If the intersection of your two total scores landed you in the **Illness Risk** section, your risk for developing an illness next year is moderately high. If you found your total scores putting you in the **High Illness Risk** section, your chance of near-future illness is high. Landing in the **Emergency** section signals the urgent need to immediately seek medical and/or psychological help!

Hopefully, your two total scores placed you in the **Wellness** or the **High Level Wellness** categories of the graph. Your risk for near future illness is then low to very low. Very likely you will remain in good health over the next year. Somewhat tongue-in-cheek, I labeled the category for extremely elevated coping with essentially no life stress as **Boredom**. I've rarely seen anyone land in this category.

You Can Now Measure Your Resilience

Resilience is present in your life when your Total Coping Score is larger than your Total Stress Score. To estimate your degree of resilience, subtract your Stress Total from your Coping Total. If the number you get is from 1 to 3, you have *Fair Resilience*. If the number is from 4 to 6, you have *Good Resilience*. A number from 7 to 10 indicates *Excellent Resilience*. I seldom see a number higher than 10. *The higher your resilience number, the lower your risk for near-future illness!*

What If Total Stress Is Greater Than Total Coping?

If your Total Stress Score is higher than your Total Coping Score, subtract your Total Coping Score from your Total Stress Score and see what number you obtain. Numbers from 1 to 3 indicate being *Mild to Moderately Out of Balance*. Numbers from 4 to 6 indicate being *Significantly Out of Balance*. Numbers from 7 to 10 indicate being *Severely Out of Balance*. When I see numbers higher than 10, it is usually an individual making a plea for help. That is, they are feeling so overwhelmed by stresses in their lives, they want someone to recognize their suffering and come to their aid immediately!

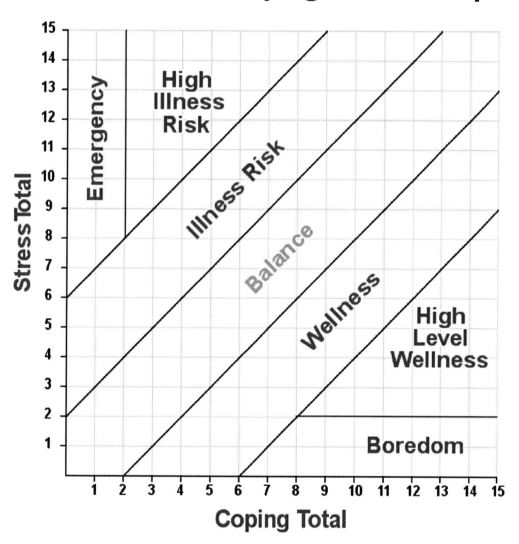

Figure 7

Further Information

Rahe, R.H., Taylor, C.B., Tolles, R.T., Newhall, L.M., Veach, T.V., and Bryson, S. A novel stress and coping workplace program reduces illness and health care utilization. Psychosomatic. *Psychosomatic Medicine*, 64:278-286, 2002.

Veach, T.L., Rahe, R.H., Tolles, R.L. and Newhall, L.M. Effectiveness of an intensive stress intervention workshop for senior managers. *Stress and Health*, 19:257-264, 2003.

Rahe, R.H. Coping and stress: a lens and filter model. Chapter in: G. Fink (Ed). *Encyclopedia of Stress* (Revised). Elsevier, pp 388-391, 2007.

Summary

If you made it this far, you have shown commendable persistence and tenacity—qualities that can lead to the achievement of several stress and coping goals presented in this book. Let's review some high points from each chapter.

Did you develop an understanding of the several sources of origin for your Strength of Character from the corresponding exercise in Chapter 1 **Who You Are**? The more biological and biographical assets you have, the better prepared you are to succeed when facing life's challenges throughout your lifetime. Remember, *success with challenge* leads to further successes. Even if you identified several biological and biographical liabilities, remember that many of these can be modified through beginning several healthy emotions and behaviors you came across in other chapters of this book, such as Behaviors and Emotions and Health Habits.

The stressful effects of a build-up of **Recent Life Changes**, particularly life changes of high intensities, may have come as a surprise to many people. This is especially true for persons who pride themselves on how many different challenges they can take on at one time in life, such as "multitaskers." But you learned from this chapter that a large number of life changes, or a few very severe life changes, can make your body prone to subsequent physical and/or psychological illnesses. As you discovered in later chapters, having coping capabilities that are greater in strength than your life changes stress can give you the resilience you need to stay healthy.

The following two chapters, **Physical Symptoms** and **Psychological Symptoms**, allowed you see if your recent life changes total points were associated with elevated physical and/

or psychological symptoms. Remember, if you had a low recent life changes total, it is very likely you also recorded few to no illness symptoms. You also learned about two categories of life stress. These were *precipitating* life stresses—as seen with high life changes stress leading to illness over the following year, and *predisposing* life stress such as the negative childhood stresses such as child abuse, which will increase illness vulnerability over a lifetime.

The last stress chapter, **Behaviors and Emotions**, might have alerted you to a previously unrecognized areas of life stress. Many persons have Type A behaviors and emotions, but they rarely see this behavior pattern in themselves. Type C behaviors and emotions included over-giving and over-caring of others, but not caring for themselves. Reptilian brain behaviors and emotions help soldiers stay alive in battle. On returning home, the reptilian brain needs to be inhibited by the frontal lobe of the new brain in order to reestablish a comfortable and productive life in civilization.

What was your **Total Stress Score**? If it was from 0 to 7 points your Stress Total was in the low to moderate range, and you probably reported few to no illness symptoms. Scores between 8 and 11 points are moderately high Stress Totals and likely to be associated with some minor illness symptoms. Total Stress Scores from 12 to 15 are very high and are nearly always associated with severe physical and psychological symptoms.

It's time to recall your coping! High **Total Stress Scores** can be balanced by equally high, and higher, **Total Coping Scores**! When stress and coping are balanced near-future illnesses are infrequent. Let's review the chapters on coping.

Were you like many persons who have very few **Health Habits**? Did you make a list of habits from chapter 6 that you plan to improve soon? Do you recall how working on the single health habit of physical fitness can result in improvements in body fat, muscle tone, diet and stopping smoking? That's four for one!

SUMMARY

The **Social Support** exercise in Chapter 7 should have been an eye-opener! Did you ever previously count your number of best friends? Have you noticed that women are better than men in developing and maintaining plentiful social support. If you are a man, find a woman to help you out, as it has been shown that when an older married man dies, his wife utilizes her close friends for support and lives on for many more productive years. Sadly, when an older married woman dies, her husband frequently becomes isolated—unless he was lucky enough to have a daughter living close by. Even then, a widower seldom has a group of supportive men to turn to and often dies shortly after the death his wife. So men, listen up!

Chapter 8, the **Responses to Stress** chapter, is a favorite of mine as I have been fortunate as a doctor to be assigned as a medical researcher and therapist for men and women surviving extremely stressful life situations. Much of what I presented in this chapter are lessons I learned from persons succeeding with enormous life challenges. You probably recognized how biological and biographical assets, combined with social support, health habits, and purpose and connection (the final coping chapter) combine to pull these persons through. You had the opportunity to examine your own problem solving abilities, your use of social support, your avoidance of exaggerated self-blame, and to learn how to improve your future stress responses to challenging life situations.

What makes you want to get up in the morning? **Life Satisfactions** do. Did you find some areas of satisfaction that helped you balance out other areas that provided very little to no satisfactions? From the additional areas of potential life satisfactions provided in this chapter, perhaps you selected one or two to give a try? A test question as to how you are doing in this area is the following: "How often do you feel absolute joy?" Persons with high life satisfactions say: "Frequently." Persons with very stressful lives, and few life satisfactions, when asked this question they often answered: "Maybe once or twice a year." Don't let that be you!

What makes life worth living? This is the theme of my final coping chapter, **Purpose and Connection**. It should be obvious to you now that I believe connecting with and helping others, especially those less fortunate than we are, is an extremely beneficial coping activity. It could even lead to some feelings of joy! In addition to frequently important religious beliefs, spirituality can also include fostering connections with others and even with the Earth. Did any of the suggested additional purpose and connections pathways give you any new ideas and plans?

What was your **Total Coping Score**? As with **Total Stress Scores**, 0 to 7 is low to moderate coping, 8 to 11 is high coping, and scores from 12 to 15 are extremely high coping. Once you obtained your **Stress and Coping Total Scores**, you were able to plot them on the **Stress and Coping Relationship Graph**? Into which section of the graph did your two total scores fall? Did your **Total Coping Score** equal or exceed your **Total Stress Score**? Remember, the greater your Total Coping compared to your Total Stress the higher is your resilience number! The higher your resilience number the less likely you are to develop any physical and psychological illnesses over the following year.

Permissions

Figure 2.

Adapted, by permission, from Donald A. Tubesing, *Structured Exercises in Stress Management*, Vol. 4, (Duluth, MN: Whole Persons Associates, Inc., © 1988, 1994).

Figures 3, 4, and 6.

Reprinted, by permission, from John M. McGrath, *Prisoner of War: Six Years in Hanoi*, (Annapolis, MD: Naval Institute Press, © 1975).

Group Instructions

This *Paths to Health and Resilience* workbook can profitably be used for group education. The workbook can be divided into 5 individual sessions where one stress indicator and one coping indicator are chosen for each session. For example, the first **Stress Indicator** (Who You Are) and the first **Coping Indicator** (Health Habits) could comprise the first session.

Before these sessions begin, however, an additional meeting is needed to make introductions of therapists and participants, to outline the goals of treatment, and to emphasize the need for both therapists and participants to carefully read the stress and coping indicators selected for each upcoming session prior to their arrivals.

Group size can be as few as 6 to 8 individuals to as many as 14 to 16 persons. It is extremely important that one or two therapists shape group discussions to follow the material presented in *Paths to Health and Resilience*.   During these discussions participants should be encouraged to relate to one another how this material applies, or does not apply, to their experiences. In this way participants become important helpers to other group members while the therapists should chiefly be facilitators for these discussions.

It is recommended that sessions be scheduled for 90 minutes in length. This allows an initial 15 to 20 minutes for latecomers to arrive as well as 10 to 15 minutes for review of participants' progress since their last meeting. The group then has at least 60 minutes remaining for a full review of their reading and important discussions of its relevance and potential applications.

At the end of each session, participants should write down one or two areas of stress management and/or coping enhancement that they commit to practicing over the time before the next session. Therefore, a small notebook should be provided for each participant that allows him or her to record their chosen practices and to document later their successes or difficulties. A review of participants' practices should be carried out over the first 15 to 20 minutes of the next 90-minute session.

Richard H. Rahe, M.D.

Professor of Psychiatry

President, Health Assessment Programs, Inc.

4543891

Made in the USA
Lexington, KY
04 February 2010